Reinventing Supermom

Support, Encouragement and Strategies for New Mothers Who Feel Lost

Kate Kripke, LCSW, PMH-C

Farfallina Press

Kate Kripke, LCSW
Founder, Director, Senior Psychotherapist
The Postpartum Wellness Center/Boulder
www.pwcboulder.com
www/katekripke.com

Published by

Farfallina Press

MLG & Associates, LLC
Princeton, NJ, 08540
www.mlgpubgroup.com

Book Design by Sheri Potter
Illustrations by Bridger Kripke
Edited by Marie Galastro

ISBN: 978-1-7360210-0-2
Printed in the United States of America

DEDICATION

To all of the incredibly brave, inspiring, and devoted mothers who have invited me into their lives during this life-changing transition called motherhood. You have all taught me more than you could possibly know. I love you all.

ENDORSEMENTS

"Kate Kripke's book is such a gift for pregnant and postpartum people! It is warm, honest, informative, and so relatable. It feels like you're talking and learning from a good friend, a great therapist, and a compassionate coach all in one place. This guide truly helps the reader know that there is a whole lot of normal in how confusing and distressing new motherhood can be, and there are lots of reliable ways to find your way through difficult times. I am grateful that this encouraging book exists in the world. As Kate says, "While being a mother is wonderful, it is also complicated. Let's make room for both, no matter how far into the journey of motherhood you are."

~ WENDY N DAVIS, PhD, PMH-C Executive Director, Postpartum Support International

"*Reinventing Supermom* is a brilliant companion for moms to take along with them for the unexpected, often exhilarating, sometimes terrifying ride of motherhood. Kate Kripke's voice is one of great confidence and comfort. She seems to know exactly what new moms need and want to hear. Her expertise shines through each page, along with her deep compassion and longstanding dedication to her work. Every single woman should have Kate Kripke by her side when navigating the challenges of new motherhood."

~ KAREN KLEIMAN, The Postpartum Stress Center, Author of "Good Moms Have Scary Thoughts" and numerous books on postpartum depression and anxiety

"As mothers, it is so easy to let our thoughts and fears take control. Through Kate Kripke's voice, guidance, and nurturing, we learn that we do have strength and hope. In this book, we discover how to move past the layers of motherhood's knots and tangles and discover the sacredness of heart-centered mothering."

- JULIE SOLOMON, Business Mentor, Best-Selling Author of Get What You Want: How to Go From Unseen to Unstoppable and Mom of two

"Kate Kripke's *Reinventing Supermom* is a gift to all of us, it's the maternal handbook you wish you had and one you can gift to everyone you know. Truthfully thoughtful and supported data, gathered from years of conversations with mothers, families and caregivers, Kripke collects it all so you no longer feel alone in the caverns of motherhood. If reading chapter to chapter or random sections when needed, this book will serve you "in the moment" or prepare you for what may lay ahead."

-KELLY COPE RUSSACK, Mom of two

TABLE OF CONTENTS

INTRODUCTION

What is this book about, why is it for me, and how do I use it?

Defining "Mom"

For the purpose of this book, a "mom" is defined as:

Any individual who considers themselves to be in the full or part-time role of nurturer, caretaker, influencer, dryer of tears, provider of hugs, holder of memories, and keeper of safety.

Foster moms, non-birth moms, adoptive moms, gender-fluid moms, and transgender moms are all included. Of course.

If you don't choose the language of "mom" but another descriptive term for your role, this book is for you, too.

In addition, while much of the language in this book uses the pronouns she/her/hers, the terms mom and mother, the image of female anatomy, and the female stereotype, and mentions dads as co-parents, I acknowledge and honor that moms and families come in many shapes and sizes, gender identities, sexual orientations, family systems, and labels.

Everyone deserves to feel well.

HOW TO USE THIS BOOK

USE IT YOUR WAY

This book is intended to give you hope, help you to feel connected, help you to find your way, and maybe even bring you joy and laughter (with some tears along the way). It contains short, simple, manageable chapters that you can access in quick bites even when you have limited attention available. Read and reread the pieces that call to you; block out the ones that don't. Get out your favorite pen and underline and highlight. Dog-ear pages. Bring it with you into the bathroom when you carve out alone time for a bath and let it get wet. It will dry. Pass it along to a friend when you are finished reading it, or store it someplace precious so that you will know where to find it when you need it most. This book is for you in whatever way makes the most sense to you. Make it yours.

A ROCKY START TO MOTHERHOOD?

You are not alone. And this book is here to help. As moms, we are told all the time—by family, neighbors, media, and the messages of commercialism—that having a baby is the happiest time of our lives. We will glow, feel blissful, and spend romantic hours in the sunlight nursing our sweet and peaceful bundles of joy.

But is it?

And will we?

Having a baby will, hopefully, bring moments of joy and connection, but it is also a time of great stress and strain on our bodies, our thinking, and our relationships. Every new mother—across all races, cultures, education levels, economics, and locations—will feel this stress and strain. This stress and strain come with the territory, but we don't talk about them enough. We don't send women into motherhood with the information that it will be hard and that reaching out for help and community is an imperative part of the postpartum journey and maternal health. Mothers need support and community to be healthy in this journey, and asking for and receiving support and help is important, necessary, and brave.

While every mother will feel the stress and strain of new parenthood, as many as 20 percent will go on to develop pregnancy-related depression or anxiety. Pregnancy-related depression and anxiety occur when a mom's brain chemistry (impacted by the shift in hormones that occurs after childbirth) and external stress combine to form a perfect storm. We consider perinatal mood and anxiety disorder to be a biological, psychological, and social dilemma.

But the good news is that moms don't have to suffer alone. There is help and support out there, just a phone call, computer screen, or car drive away. There are books, like this one, that can help you gain the motivation and spirit you need to get unstuck. As the founding director of the Postpartum Wellness Center/Boulder and a psychotherapist specializing in reproductive mental health, I talk with moms every day about ways to feel better in motherhood. Moms who are supported biologically, psychologically, and socially are less likely to suffer from depression and anxiety and are more likely to have a healthy emotional adjustment to motherhood.

And so, to you, Dear Mama, welcome. Welcome to the first step (or maybe it's one of your many steps!) in finding relief from this all-out chaotic start to your journey. You made it here. You picked up this book. You opened it. You started to read. You are on your road to wellness.

IF WONDER WOMAN WAS A MOTHER

If Wonder Woman was a mother, she would have wider hips and a softer belly and breasts that drooped. And she would still wear that badass outfit.

If Wonder Woman was a mother, you would find Cheerios in her hair underneath her perfect curls and raisins in her fingernails underneath her bright red nail polish.

If Wonder Woman was a mother, her curls wouldn't be perfect, really. Her hair would be thrown together without a mirror, or, perhaps, her Wonder Woman locks would be styled by her children with bright red, plastic barrettes. She would still look beautiful.

If Wonder Woman was a mother, her superpower would be to take the edge off pain simply by saying, "I'm here."

If Wonder Woman was a mother, her Wonder Woman bracelets would have the power to fill a heart, to grow one's faith in themself, to help someone feel safe and secure in their own skin.

If Wonder Woman was a mother, she would proudly acknowledge her imperfections. She would stand firmly on her two feet, her arms down by her sides with her palms facing forward, and her head held high. She would look the world in the eye and say, "Yes. This is Me! I am messy and uncertain and unsure of myself from time to time. And I am proud."

If Wonder Woman was a mother, she would embody a tender heart underneath all of that bravery. She would be scared much of the time. Yes, scared. And she would keep on going anyway. Which would make her even braver.

If Wonder Woman was a mother, she would have a therapist. Obviously.

If Wonder Woman was a mother, she would model boundaries like a badass. She would say no without apology. She would stop helping others when what she needed most was to help herself. She would fill herself up whenever she could so that she could continue to save the world. But she would know, people. She would know to put her oxygen mask on first.

If Wonder Woman was a mother, she would sit quietly every day, before she descended on the bad guys, and she would reflect. She would invite in her discomfort and become really familiar with it so that she never needed to run away from the shit that she didn't like. Wonder Woman never runs away, of course, but that comes from some serious practice.

If Wonder Woman was a mother, she would know the difference between a situation that needed accepting and a problem that needed fixing. This Wonder Woman would know how to reserve her energy. In this Wonder Woman's world, there aren't really as many problems out there as one might think. This Wonder Woman's biggest superpower is acceptance.

If Wonder Woman was a mother, I would immediately re-establish my 1970s obsession with superheroes. I would put all my eggs in her basket. I would feel forever safe and accepted and protected from the bad guys (who often live in my head like they do for the rest of you, but, well, she would figure that out too).

If Wonder Woman was a mother, well, she would be all the more wonder-full.

Because she would be real.

I. FACTS:
Data & Research

The Difference between Postpartum Depression and Healthy New Mom Stress

Postpartum depression may be common, but it's not normal. Baby blues is common and normal. So what's the difference between baby blues and postpartum depression?

Suffering in new motherhood is not normal. Feeling anxious most of the time is not normal. Feeling overwhelmed most of the time is not normal, and feeling trapped and angry and uncertain most of the time is not normal. Motherhood is overwhelming and scary for most of us, but when these feelings take charge—when they become more dominant than feelings of relative well-being—something else is going on.

I get my feathers ruffled every time I hear a new mother say that their friend, family member, or doctor told them that the distress they are feeling is just part of being a new mom. Yes, being a new mom is complicated and hard and distressing at times, but I am concerned each time a mom says that she waited to get help for postpartum depression because she just assumed that the way she was feeling came with new motherhood, or that she just had to get used to the suffering, or that the pain would go away on its own. I become furious when I read articles or blog entries that assume postpartum depression is caused by a woman's resistance to all that comes with motherhood. Frankly, it's all BS. I want to yell this from the treetops.

So, here, my friends, is a bit of a reminder for all of you, and perhaps something to use as a guide if you are not so sure whether the way you are feeling needs outside support. Here's how to tell the difference between "normal" new mom stress and postpartum depression:

Healthy New Mom Adjustment

- Some feelings of being overwhelmed and anxious, that decrease with reassurance
- Some "escapist fantasies" (a desire to run away) that occur when the logistics of mothering are challenging, but go away when your baby is soothed, when you are rested, and when you are validated
- Fears about harm coming to your baby that come and go, that you know are not "realistic" and that do not cause lasting distress, and that decrease as your experience and comfort with motherhood grow
- Sleeplessness that occurs from caring for your baby at night, while still having the ability to sleep when your baby is sleeping or when given the option to rest
- Fatigue that comes from late-night feedings and interrupted sleep
- Some feelings of frustration toward your partner regarding differences in parenting choices or differing roles
- Moments of sadness, disappointment, or anger toward your parents when reminded of the ways that you were parented, but the ability to hold insight and perspective regarding your own relationship with your baby
- Feelings of isolation that are caused by the increased time spent with your baby, especially a newborn, but also a desire and motivation to connect with others
- Uncertainty that comes with this new job, and building confidence that comes with time
- A hesitancy and worry that comes with allowing others to care for your baby, but a willingness to do this when you are in need of a break
- A decrease in eating that is caused by the logistics of being a new mom
- Temporary body aches and pains that are a result of childbirth and/or breastfeeding
- Feelings of worry about your baby's ability to latch or feed as you hoped that decrease with feeding improvement, or that shift when a new feeding option is chosen

- Acknowledgment of the challenge that comes with new motherhood, but also the ability to look forward to things getting easier
- Increases in energy that come with increases in sleep
- Vulnerable feelings that come and go but that do not alter the way you think about yourself

Postpartum Distress That Requires Support

- Feeling anxious and overwhelmed most of the time, an anxiety that doesn't go away with reassurance
- Feelings of regret over becoming a mom that do not seem to go away
- Repetitive and intrusive thoughts of harm coming to your baby that cause great distress and that impact your ability to care for your baby
- Thoughts of hurting yourself
- Sleeplessness that occurs due to "monkey brain"— anxious thoughts that will not go away
- A deep fatigue that is not alleviated with rest and/or a desire to remain in bed all day
- Lack of appetite or a need to keep eating despite being full
- Body aches and pains with no apparent cause
- Relentless feelings of anger or rage toward your partner and/or others
- Resurfacing memories about your own early childhood that cause great distress, anxiety, or sadness
- Loneliness and isolation that occur while also pulling away from those who care about you; a lack of desire or motivation to connect with others
- Persistent feelings that you're not a good mom or you're not good at doing motherly things, even despite validation or reassurance from others
- Feelings that your baby does not "like" you because he cries or is not feeding well
- Unrelenting anxiety about having others help care for your baby and a deep fear and inability to let go of some of this control
- Never-ending feelings that you will never feel better
- Sudden increase in energy that occurs despite a decrease in sleep; this may or may not include seeing or hearing things that aren't really there
- A general feeling of "not feeling like yourself"

- Any uncomfortable or vulnerable feelings that persist for longer than two to three weeks, especially when these interfere with your ability to meet your basic needs and/or live your life as you would like to

Please remember, moms, new motherhood is challenging for all of us, but motherhood should not be consistently distressing or miserable. If you are finding yourself wondering if what you are struggling with is "normal," a good question to ask yourself is: *"Is this normal for me when I am well?"* If not, there is help waiting. You do not need to suffer through postpartum depression.

If you are a new mom who is not necessarily experiencing symptoms of depression and anxiety but is struggling in this new chapter of your life, welcome to the club! I have yet to meet a new mom who easily coasts through this stage of life. But first-time moms who don't have the necessary skills to tolerate the discomfort that comes with motherhood will more likely experience some degree of suffering if they don't make the commitment to true, deep self-care.

If you have this book in your hands, you are telling me that you strive to be a healthy mother, both physically, psychologically, and socially. You want to be all you can be for your children. This book will give you the tools to start on the path to wellness that all new mothers need.

I am thrilled that you are here, ready to start your journey toward being a healthy, happy, and loving mother.

What Is "Postpartum Depression" Anyway?

Postpartum depression (PPD) and anxiety are usually the last things you are thinking about when you both muddle and dance through the nine or so months of your pregnancy. You've likely heard about PPD before in the news, or perhaps your midwife or OB has mentioned it to you, but my guess is that for the most part, the idea of these very unfortunate happenings kind of goes in one ear and out the other. PPD is surrounded by myths that we all know and quiver at anyway: *If you have PPD, it means that you want to hurt yourself or your baby. If you say you have PPD, someone will take your baby away. If you are not happy in early motherhood, you must be a terrible mother. If you are depressed or anxious during pregnancy or early motherhood, you should just plow through and get over it.* With these myths (and yes, they are all myths, but more on that later), who on Earth would want to consider being affiliated with anything like postpartum depression?

But here is the thing: Perinatal Mood Disorders (occurring during pregnancy and/or postpartum and including PPD) are pretty darn common. In fact, about one in five new mothers will struggle with some form of depression and/or anxiety sometime during pregnancy or during the first 12 months after having a baby. Guess what? Moms with postpartum depression and anxiety are really no different than you and me. These women are professors, artists, lawyers, athletes, students, cooks, writers. They are labor and delivery nurses, pediatricians, obstetricians, and midwives. They are librarians, teachers, accountants. They are mothers, wives, partners, friends. They are human. They are creative. They are witty and wise. These women are thinkers. They are dreamers. They love to laugh. They often cry. These women are bold. They are brave. And they are beautiful.

As my late colleague Bill Myer at Duke University once stated:

These are mothers in strained relationships with the baby's fathers, or those dealing with the added stress of an unconventional lifestyle. These are the mothers with careers who always wanted to be mothers but now, at home, miss the challenges and adult stimulation of their former employments. They are the working mothers who out of necessity had to return too soon to work and had to leave their babies in less-than-optimal child-care. They are the relocated mothers who just moved to the area due to their partners' job transfers and find themselves alone in an unfamiliar city. They are the anxious mothers of hard-to-soothe babies. They are the perfectionist mothers who have always held themselves to impossibly high standards and now as new mothers feel they are failures. They are the mothers who were used to having a fair amount of control over their lives until they had early deliveries, unexpected C-sections, or babies with special needs. They are the giving mothers whose babies have colic, won't sleep, won't take the breast, and won't be consoled. They are hard on themselves, sleep-deprived, and even food-deprived.

These women are highly competent and well-loved. They just also happen to be struggling at a time when they least expected or wanted to.

Postpartum mood or anxiety disorders like postpartum depression are the most common complication of childbirth. They are also a complication that most new mothers do not expect. Within 24 hours of childbirth, estrogen and progesterone drop dramatically, and this hormonal shift has a direct impact on brain chemistry. While the vulnerability in brain chemistry will resolve within about 2-3 weeks for about 80% new mothers, the remaining 20% of mothers will continue to have a vulnerable brain chemistry that makes them less resilient to the biological, psychological, and social stressors that accompany new motherhood. Lacking sleep, nutrition depletion, dehydration, physical healing from childbirth, birth trauma, breast feeding challenges, identity shifts, the huge responsibility of caring for a newborn, relationship conflicts including early childhood trauma, major life changes postpartum, and isolation can all lead to symptoms of depression and anxiety for a new mom who is now less resilient to stress. The biggest takeaway from this? PPD is not a woman's fault and has absolutely nothing to do with the kind of mother that she is or wants to be.

It is important that these moms get the support they need and deserve. Because while PPD does not mean that you are a terrible mother, it does make it difficult to enjoy the early weeks and months of parenting and may interfere with your ability to bond and attach with your baby.

The raw truth is that having a new baby is not easy for anyone, no matter what kind of "perfect" they appear to be from the outside. We all struggle, each and every one of us. But those of us whose struggle outweighs the happiness and hopefulness needed to care for a new baby need not feel this way. Help is available. Asking for it is usually the hardest part.

A SUMMARY OF PPD FACTS

- If a mom struggles emotionally in the first months or years after giving birth, she is "in good company." Approximately 20 percent of women who give birth will have some form of PPD.
- The most common symptom of PPD is ANXIETY, not depression.
- Normal baby-blues symptoms should subside within two to three weeks. If a mom continues to feel sad, lonely,

overwhelmed, emotionally vulnerable, unable to sleep when her baby is sleeping, unable to make decisions, irritable, hopeless, anxious despite reassurance, and unlike herself after two to three weeks, she should consider talking to a professional and/or seeking other forms of support.

- PPD is treatable! Supports that have helped many women get through symptoms of PPD include exercise, therapy, medication, acupuncture, community and support groups, yoga and meditation, nutrition, and sleep.
- The sooner a mom gets support for symptoms of PPD, the sooner she will feel like herself again and the less severe these symptoms will become.
- Sleep deprivation is known to be a major factor in the development of PPD. Getting at least four hours of uninterrupted sleep a night is a great way to be proactive in the prevention of PPD. How? Enlist the help of friends and family, make a plan to share nighttime feedings with your spouse/partner, or enlist the help of a doula or night nanny.
- Some relatively simple ways to prevent symptoms of PPD include: easy to moderate exercise including yoga, healthy nutrition, adequate sleep, finding a moms' group or support network, getting fresh air, staying hydrated, talking to friends/spouse about how you feel, and deep breathing and/or meditation exercises.
- When a woman struggles with PPD, it is not her fault or a reflection of how much she loves her baby. It does, how ever, disturb her ability to enjoy the early weeks and months of parenthood.
- It is important for every mom to take care of herself physically as well as emotionally because PPD and other adjustment issues may affect the physical and emotional development of her baby if they are not treated appropriately.

- Some risk factors that make it more likely that a mom might suffer from PPD include:

  ~ A previous history of depression, anxiety, or other mental health challenges

  ~ Symptoms of, or treatment for, depression, anxiety, or other mental health challenges during pregnancy

  ~ Inadequate social support

  ~ Severe premenstrual syndrome (PMS) or premenstrual dysphoric disorder (PMDD) prior to becoming pregnant

  ~ Major life changes before or during pregnancy or following childbirth (move, death of a loved one, loss of a job, marital conflict)

  ~ Unwanted pregnancy

What Maternal Anxiety Looks and Feels Like

One in five mothers reading this will be able to relate to all or some of what is written here about maternal anxiety. 20 percent. If you, personally, aren't struggling with anxiety, then I promise you some mother that you know is.

What does maternal anxiety look and feel like?

- It looks like an inability to sit still; an agitated need to do something, anything, to not sit still.
- It looks like tossing and turning in the night; exhausted, sleepless hours spent thinking about all of the things that could go wrong.
- It looks like calls to the pediatrician, Google searches late into the night, too-frequent checks on the baby or kiddo (even when the baby or kiddo is quiet and sleeping soundly).
- It looks like asking for reassurance. But then still needing more. But never actually getting what you are looking for.
- It feels like jumpiness, agitation, fast heart rates, and quick breaths.
- It feels like pain, sometimes. Back pain or headaches, or neck pain, or jaw pain, or stomach pain, or sometimes just pain that is totally indescribable.
- It feels like frustration or irritability or anger or even rage.
- It feels like dying, sometimes.

Maternal anxiety feeds off the *not knowing*, the *uncertainty*, and the *inability to control* the things we want to control (like eating and sleeping and crying and total 100 percent safety all the time). Sometimes the feelings of deep, underlying discomfort (no, let's actually call it pain) are so huge that you can't tolerate being with it at all, and so your brain—your thinking—jumps in to try to figure out how to make the feelings go away: Cue in the obsessive and addictive behavior like the cleaning or the Google searching or the problem-solving or the assessing the potential danger or the drinking or the round-and-round-and-round-she-goes monkey braining that we call ruminating thoughts and obsessive thinking.

I don't know if you have ever considered this, but it is an important point for reflection: *Did you know that your anxiety stems from a deep-rooted fear of pain and death and loss? That all of that anxious thinking is fueled up by your terror of uncertainty and unpredictability and your fear of losing this thing that you now love more than anything that you have ever had?*

Attachment and grief are connected at the hip. The more we allow ourselves to love, the more pain we feel if that thing goes away. So, for many of you, you distract yourself with the thinking and planning and trying to control so that you don't have to slow down and just be and connect deeply with the love that you feel for this little human. The anxiety and the obsessions are the buffer. They serve a purpose of distracting you from the depth of your love and pain, because you fear that those feelings are too powerful for you. But the catch? If you aren't willing to feel the discomfort and pain of uncertainty, you will not feel the depths of your love in all of its beauty. You can't have one without the other. They come together, and you either get both of them or neither.

The anxiety stops when the bolting from the reality of uncertainty stops. The obsessive behavior stops when the trying to escape from the reality of what is right here stops. I know, it sounds unrealistic and impossible and probably annoying. But it's true. I know because I have been there. This is also my study and my work, and I see this over and over and over in the women whom I support every day.

So, if you are one of those one in five mothers who is nodding along or tearing up or taking a deep breath to find some air, I see you. We see you.

Pause. Feel your feet on the floor. Really, right now: Pause and feel your feet on the floor. Take a big, deep breath—the biggest breath you've taken yet today. Feel the air on your skin, the floor underneath your feet, the seat underneath you. Notice what you hear. What you smell.

And then answer this question:

Right now—right in this moment with your feet on this floor and the air on your skin and this seat underneath you—are you okay?

I thought so. Yes, in this moment. Right now. You are okay!

Each time you do that and ask yourself that question, you will find the same answer. Every. Single. Time.

In this moment, you are okay.

What Maternal Depression Looks and Feels Like

Sometimes it hits hard and out of the blue.

Sometimes it is a slow unraveling that occurs over time.

Either way, it feels like being trapped in the darkness of a long tunnel with no visible way out.

Depression can suck away all of your energy and motivation and curiosity and hope. Simply getting out of bed, brushing your teeth, combing your hair, and making breakfast can feel like an impossible journey.

"What's the point?" and *"Everything is too hard"* can feel like the only phrases accessible to your depressed brain.

Depression calls the shots. Other people are confused by the deep hole that someone who is depressed is in. They try to call to you at the bottom. They get frustrated that you can't hear them. They try to throw you a rope but don't understand that even lifting your arms to reach toward the offer is too exhausting. Pretty soon their care turns to frustration. You feel their anger, but nobody understands that what you both share is deep fear that you will never emerge from the distant darkness.

Sometimes you cry without understanding why. Your tears flow without intent or control. Sadness is the only emotion you know.

Sometimes all you feel is pain—in your bones, in your skin, in your head, in your belly. The pain is physical and sharp and never-ending.

Sometimes you feel nothing at all. You are numb to everything and feel like you move through the motions without even knowing that you are there experiencing it all.

Your baby cries out. Your child reaches for your hand. Your teenager comes and goes, and whichever stage of mothering you are in, you are unable to respond at all. You no longer know how. You feel lost in your own darkness and can't imagine how to be a human, let alone a parent.

It's all too much.

This is what depression can feel like. If you are a new mother, please know that one in every five of you reading this is in the boat. If you are a mother with children older than one, please know that one in every 10 of you reading this is in the boat with you.

You are not alone. Even though you could swear that you are.

Please don't give up the small efforts at reaching for the rope and beginning the climb out. Today and tomorrow and the next day, do one thing that feels impossible but also begins the climb: *Step out into the sunshine. Eat an apple. Pet your dog. Wash your face. Take a long, deep breath. Make a call. Let someone know that you need help.*

The only way out of depression is through the deep feelings of despair and grief and hurt. Pain always needs attention. Your feelings always make sense. Feelings and emotions matter and they are wise beyond belief. They are here to teach you how to love yourself more fully, and once you learn how to do this, you will begin to feel better. I know, it feels impossible, doesn't it? But I promise it's not, and when you begin to access that acceptance and love, the sun will begin to shine again. That's just how it works.

15 Myths about Pregnancy, Birth, and Postpartum

Oh, yes ma'am. Pregnancy, birth, and postpartum are surrounded by many myths. Too many. So, let's take a minute to debate some widely held beliefs about Postpartum Depression and other Postpartum Mood Disorders. It's about time.

MYTH #1: When you are pregnant, you will feel better than you have ever felt. In fact, you will glow!

FACT: While some women describe pregnancy as wonderfully full—a time when they felt more energetic than ever, when they felt the glow that others commented on daily, and when they felt happy and alive—this is not, actually, the norm. Most women go through stages of incredible difficulty during their pregnancies. Many women feel uncharacteristically fatigued and irritable. Many women feel more exhausted than they imagined they would feel. Many women feel nauseated throughout the nine-plus months when they share their bodies with their little ones. Many women never, actually, "glow" and instead feel deeply depleted. I need not remind you, Dear Readers, that even the women who most detest being pregnant love their babies to pieces. And, if you do happen to be one of those women who love pregnancy, that is awesome! The many women who do not can borrow some of that energy from you.

MYTH #2: Feeling anxious and overwhelmed is just a part of pregnancy and postpartum, and moms should just get used to this.

FACT: While it is absolutely true that all women can expect to feel anxious and overwhelmed about being pregnant and/or becoming a parent, this does not mean that women need to suffer through these periods. While not every pregnant mom needs therapeutic support, most women who are pregnant will benefit from reaching out to others when they feel this way. Having the space to talk about your feelings and conflicts is incredibly important for the wellness of every woman, and by no means do women simply need to push through periods of vulnerability.

MYTH #3: Women's bodies are made to birth babies. Women give birth all the time. Everywhere. Therefore, women should not have a need for any sort of pain support during childbirth such as an epidural.

FACT: Yes, women's bodies are made to birth babies. Yes, women do this everywhere. However, this does *not* mean that a mom should feel ashamed for asking for an epidural or other system of pain relief during her childbirth. Each woman has an absolute right to ask for what she needs throughout this process. If you happen to be a mother who used pain medication, yay to you for paying attention to what you need.

MYTH #4: It is ridiculous for women to try to birth their babies "naturally." We are a country in which many aids for pain are safe and available. Why put yourself through something you need not do?

FACT: Yes, we are fortunate to have many systems available for reduction of pain. But, again, no one fast rule exists for how women "should" choose to birth their babies. In communities where it is common to give birth to children without interventions, women succeed in this time and time again. So, if you are a mother who chose to birth her baby without pain medication? Yay, you, for doing what felt right for you.

MYTH #5: Women feel an unrelenting rush of euphoria after delivering their babies. Instantly, "mommy-ness" kicks in, and the bond and attachment happen all at once.

FACT: Well, no, not necessarily. Many women do get the wonderful opportunity to have this experience after delivery, but many, many women also feel what is described as a "delayed response" to being a mom. Some of the women who have this initial experience of uncertain emotion will go on to develop a postpartum mood or anxiety disorder, but many will not. For some women, this deep connection with their babies just takes time.

MYTH #6: Competent, high-functioning women should expect themselves to be able to handle the many emotional and logistical pieces that come with caring for a baby all on their own.

FACT: This myth both angers and amazes me—we all seem to believe this one at some level. In many cultures and communities, the idea of "it takes a village" is a literal reality for women who birth babies. In many cultures and communities, new mothers are fed, bathed, pampered, and kept in community for months after they give birth. In this way, it is expected that this new mom will be assisted by many, many others as she transitions into her new role as mama. And yet oftentimes we still find that it is an unspoken expectation that women should do this all on their own—gracefully, happily, and with total acceptance. And what happens because of this is that women become deeply disappointed in themselves when they are unable to do so. Please, no matter how high-functioning you are, don't attempt to do this alone.

MYTH #7: Breastfeeding comes naturally.

FACT: Perhaps this one is true for some women, but for most of my colleagues, friends, and clients, this is not the case. In fact, I think it is probably fair to say that breastfeeding is difficult, at least in the beginning, for *most* mothers. Be it nipple pain, difficulty in latching, over- or underproduction of milk, or difficulty in settling into a "hold" that works, many women go through significant challenges when beginning to breastfeed. Working with a lactation consultant can be valuable for many of these women. Still, some will either decide to stop or find that the challenge of breastfeeding is just too difficult to see through. There is absolutely no shame in this, and my hope is that each woman feels empowered to make a decision around breastfeeding that works best for her and her baby. Babies most certainly benefit from breast milk. But what they need even more than breast milk is their mothers.

MYTH #8: The baby blues and postpartum depression are the same thing.

FACT: Nope. Many people refer to PPD as "the blues," but these are two entirely different challenges. The baby blues affect around 85 percent of new mothers and last for no longer than two to three weeks. The baby blues are considered a "normal" part of the postpartum experience because they are so common and are a basic consequence of the shifting hormones and brain chemistry that follow birth. PPD, however, affects about 15 to 20 percent of new moms, and while symptoms may be similar to the baby blues, they can become much more serious over time. The blues usually go away on their own, while PPD usually requires professional support and treatment.

MYTH #9: All mothers are sleep deprived. All mothers are emotional. All mothers are anxious and irritable and overwhelmed. It's just part of the journey.

FACT: Yes, having a new baby makes it much more difficult to get the sleep that your body needs. Yes, transitioning to motherhood can be hugely overwhelming. However, as with myth #2, being anxious, overwhelmed, tearful, and unable to sleep most of the time is *not* a "normal" part of new motherhood. New moms can expect to have moments of all of the above, but whenever a mom finds that she is feeling this way more times than not, something else is probably going on. Too many women wait out months and months of suffering because they believe or are told that this is just the way it is and they should get used to it. This is neither true nor fair.

MYTH #10: I should just pull myself together.

FACT: Depression and anxiety are real illnesses, and you are really suffering. This does not mean that you are weak and lazy; usually this is not something that a mom can conquer on her own. Many, many moms waste months of time trying to tell themselves that they are okay, when they really are not. With adequate help, these precious months can be spent feeling more connected to your baby and feeling better about yourself.

MYTH #11: If I tell anyone how I am feeling, they will take my baby away.

FACT: Having PPD is not a reason for anyone to take your baby away. In fact, when a mom reaches out for help, we know that she is getting support not just for herself, but also for her baby, children, and partner/spouse. Support for PPD is in service of the whole family.

MYTH #12: Moms who love their children also love the responsibilities of being a mom.

FACT. Ahhhhhh. Hmmm. Nope again. The amount of love that you have for your baby has nothing to do with the amount of love (or patience) that you have for dirty diapers at 4 a.m., bouncing and rocking all hours of the day, breastfeeding with bleeding nipples, and trying hour after hour to soothe a baby who seems unable to be soothed. Love your baby all you want, moms. But please, please, please work hard not to judge yourselves if you are having a difficult time transitioning into this new role. Simply put, it is hard.

MYTH #13: Nobody understands.

FACT: I know that it can feel this way. However, an entire army of women exists who struggle postpartum, and you just might find that when you are ready to talk about your challenges with postpartum depression or anxiety, people who have had the same experiences will come out of the woodwork. In addition, many of us involved in raising awareness about postpartum mood and anxiety disorders are training doctors, nurses, midwives, and educators all over the world so that many more appropriately informed and trained providers are there to support you.

MYTH #14: My postpartum mood disorder will ruin my baby.

FACT: While we do know that untreated or under-treated perinatal mood and anxiety disorders (PMADs) can have lasting negative effects on infant and child development, we also know that women who do seek help get well—and their babies thrive along with them. As you learn more about how to take good care of yourself, find happiness, and be more present, your little ones will reap the benefits. You may just find that your postpartum challenges, once treated, actually lead to more present, healthy, and happy children. When you are your best, they will most likely be too.

MYTH #15: There are no safe treatments, so why bother getting help?

FACT: Many excellent, safe, and effective treatments exist for PPD. Many anti-depressant and anti-anxiety medications have been shown to be safe to take while pregnant and breastfeeding. Supportive treatments such as acupuncture, mild to moderate exercise, meditation and mindfulness practices, and nutritional counseling have also been shown to help relieve symptoms of depression and anxiety.

Those myths are like the bad guys we are trying to take down. Really, they only have power if you allow them to have it. Underneath it all, these myths are just made from fear.

Should You Have a Baby if You Struggle with Serious Mental Illness?

Let's say you are in the high-risk category for developing a postpartum mood or anxiety disorder like postpartum depression. You have battled depression, anxiety, OCD, or bipolar disorder throughout your lifetime, and you have been told that the major hormonal and identity shifts that occur during pregnancy and childbirth are likely to push you out of remission, aggravate your symptoms, or lead to even more mental health challenges than you have already faced, like psychosis perhaps. Maybe you are currently taking medicine, and maybe you are not. Maybe you are willing to continue your medication while pregnant, and maybe you are not. Maybe you have already had a child and suffered with severe postpartum mental illness including psychosis, and maybe you have not. But one thing is for sure: You desperately want a baby, and you are scared to death about what this might mean for you. And for your child.

These are tough questions, and anyone who identifies with the above snapshot can attest to how unbearably complicated all of this can feel. Struggling with a perinatal mood and anxiety disorder when you didn't see it coming is like a blow to the head that knocks you flat for a while. Thinking ahead and knowing that you are likely to struggle gives a mom the chance to plan ahead for support, but can also be downright terrifying.

Perinatal mental illness awareness is increasing, but the fact is that many highly skilled medical professionals are out there who still are not up to date, informed, and knowledgeable about the many elements to consider when it comes to perinatal mental health. Women are told to not even consider having children due to mental illness when there may be safe ways to do so. Women are told to stop taking their medication during pregnancy when this is neither necessary nor safe. Women are given wrong information all the time, and life-changing decisions are made without adequate information. This is a problem.

This is what we know, in no particular order:

- Moms who have struggled with depression, anxiety, OCD, bipolar disorder, and psychosis are more likely to struggle with mental illness postpartum than mothers who have not.
- Moms who have a history of bipolar disorder are 25 to 30 percent more likely to develop postpartum psychosis than moms who do not.
- No concrete evidence exists that proves pregnancy prevents mania or depression in women with bipolar disorder.
- Discontinuing medication during pregnancy opens up the possibility for relapse in women with mental illness.

- The first four to eight weeks after delivery is the most critical time for women with bipolar disorder, as this is when most cases of psychosis become evident. During this period, it is IMPERATIVE that moms get adequate sleep, nutrition, and exercise.
- Under the attentive care of a trained and appropriate medical provider, a mom who suffers severe mental illness can become pregnant and go on to deliver a healthy baby and be symptom-free.
- Whether or not to take medicine to treat symptoms of mental illness while pregnant is a question best answered under the direct care of a trained and appropriate medical provider.
- Most moms with severe symptoms of mental illness, including bipolar disorder, will require medication support during pregnancy in order to manage symptoms and/or remain symptom-free.
- Many medicines required for the treatment of mental illness including depression, anxiety, OCD, and bipolar disorder are known to be safe enough for pregnant moms when weighed against the known risk to both mom and baby of untreated or under-treated symptoms. Many, many women take these medicines while pregnant and go on to deliver healthy and thriving newborns.
- Current research tells us that, in most cases, moms with mental illness, including bipolar disorder, can absolutely have healthy pregnancies.
- Postpartum bipolar disorder and psychosis are both temporary and treatable with adequate professional help.

Women who suffer from more severe mental illness are much more likely to develop perinatal mental illness than women who do not, and without appropriate medical care, many of these women will be at a very high risk for psychosis and hospitalization. And so, what to consider if you are one of these women?

- How severe is your mental illness, and are you willing to do the work required to both prevent and treat symptoms?
- Do you have adequate support lined up, including a reproductive psychiatrist, therapist trained in perinatal mental health, understanding partner, and OB who is knowledgeable and supportive of women who need to take medicine while pregnant in order to be well?
- Will you be able to maintain adequate rest/sleep, nutrition, exercise, and stress management while pregnant and into the postpartum year, and do you have the imperative support lined up to do so in order to prevent the aggravation of symptoms?

- If you have had a child before, what supports can you put into place that may help to reduce symptoms the second time around?

This is all very personal, and while some families may decide not to get pregnant because the risk of mental illness relapse or psychosis is too high, others may feel strongly that they are willing to take these risks and do the work in order to be healthy while pregnant and caring for a baby. No matter where you are with this, the one thing that is certain is as follows: When making the decisions about whether or not to have a child if you suffer from current or previous mental illness, it will be important to understand the very imperative role that medical, therapeutic, and community support will play in your journey. Moms who have this history cannot do it alone. Nor should they need to.

Postpartum OCD: What You Need to Know

When we refer to "postpartum *depression*," we miss the ball for many, many women who struggle during pregnancy or after giving birth. Sure, tons of women become depressed during pregnancy or after (about one in five, actually), but even more women struggle with some form of anxiety, whether that be generalized anxiety, panic, obsessive-compulsive disorder (OCD), or post-traumatic stress disorder (PTSD). I can't tell you how many women wait for a very long time to call me and receive support because they "didn't have postpartum depression because they weren't depressed." In truth, postpartum depression (as opposed to general depression) is a very *anxious* depression, meaning that women not only feel depressed, but feel hugely, unbelievably, and often devastatingly anxious.

One of the postpartum anxiety disorders that women might struggle with is Postpartum obsessive-compulsive disorder (postpartum OCD). Studies suggest that three to five percent of new moms will experience symptoms of OCD, but I truly believe that the numbers are much greater than that. In my Boulder psychotherapy practice, probably two-thirds of the women whom I see are suffering from OCD symptoms. In my world, this illness is very, very common. Yet a ton of shame and guilt come along with the very common OCD symptoms, and as a result, many women are afraid to let people know that they are struggling.

And what does "struggling" mean for these moms? Moms who have postpartum OCD suffer repetitive, frequent, intrusive, and often very scary thoughts of harm coming to themselves or their babies. While not all women struggling with postpartum OCD have these characteristic scary thoughts, most of them do, and often in their thoughts they are the ones causing the harm. These thoughts are usually gruesome, disturbing, scary, and unexpected. Women who struggle with postpartum OCD say that these thoughts appear out of nowhere and that they feel they cannot control when these thoughts come and go. Moms who have these thoughts are very disturbed by the very fact that they occur. They know that the thoughts they're having are wrong, and they're confused by the fact that these thoughts have nothing to do with the ways they imagine themselves to be as mothers.

These moms will do everything they can to keep their babies safe. The "obsessions" in OCD refer to the thoughts, and the "compulsions" refer to the behaviors that accompany those thoughts in an attempt to reduce the anxiety that the thoughts create. These moms will avoid anything that makes them afraid they might hurt their babies in any way. They might avoid public places or obsessively wash baby bottles. They might hide all sharp objects in their home. They might refuse to give their babies baths, or walk down stairs while carrying their babies, or drive in a car with their babies. Frequently, when support isn't put into place, these moms will say that they feel like their babies are safer without them. We actually do not worry about moms hurting their babies when they suffer from OCD; again, we know they will do anything in their power to keep their babies safe. But we do worry about those moms who do not receive adequate support because their symptoms can become unbearable.

Let me be very clear here: *Postpartum OCD is* **NOT** *the same as* postpartum psychosis. Although every mom with OCD feels like she is on the brink of going "crazy" and fears that she will "snap" or do something to her child that she doesn't want to do, the simple reality that she has these fears and wonders if she is psychotic lets us know that she is not. Unlike women with OCD, women who suffer from postpartum psychosis (PPP) do not know that the thoughts they are having are wrong. They do not necessarily feel like they are going "crazy" because they are in their own reality that is out of touch with "right" and "wrong." Typically guilt, shame, and anxiety do not accompany the thoughts that occur with postpartum psychosis. And unfortunately, the women who suffer with PPP do not always do everything in their control to keep their babies safe from harm. (And, yet, every mom with postpartum OCD who walks into my office tells me that she is sure she is going crazy. Suddenly, every hyped-up media story about postpartum psychosis feels very close to home.)

Research tells us that up to 70 percent of women who suffer from OCD symptoms prior to becoming pregnant will have a resurgence of symptoms during their pregnancies or postpartum period. It is believed that somewhere between 13 to 59 percent of new moms who experience OCD after giving birth will be experiencing OCD for the first time; and 29 percent of those women who have suffered from OCD in their lifetime will experience an exasperation of symptoms during the postpartum year. One of the biggest risk factors in developing postpartum OCD is having a personal or family history of OCD or high-level anxiety.

The good news? (Yes, good news exists!) Postpartum OCD is absolutely treatable. As with other perinatal mood and anxiety disorders, we know that when women seek out help and follow treatment recommendations, they get well. All of them.

OCD is treated best through a combination of medication and therapy support. We know that OCD is primarily a biochemical issue, and therefore it responds well to SSRIs (selective serotonin reuptake inhibitors) and other anti-depressant and anti-anxiety medication. Usually, once a woman gets on the right medicine for balancing out her biochemistry, she will notice a relief in symptoms within a few weeks. I see it happen all the time.

Psychotherapy (especially therapy that includes cognitive behavioral strategies) helps mom to develop techniques for stress reduction and changing thought patterns that contribute to her anxiety. Therapy really helps a mom realize that she is not crazy, she is not alone, and she is, in fact, a fabulous mom to her kiddo.

So, please, if this all resonates for you or someone you know, reach out for the help you deserve.

For a great book on postpartum OCD, I recommend *Dropping the Baby and Other Scary Thoughts* by Karen Kleiman, MSW.

Some Information on Postpartum Psychosis

In my practice, I'm often asked about the differences between postpartum depression and postpartum psychosis. Let's take a moment to clarify these two terms.

While moms who have postpartum psychosis are likely to have symptoms of depression and anxiety, postpartum psychosis is considered a different mental health diagnosis than postpartum depression and postpartum anxiety. Postpartum depression is known to affect approximately 20 percent of women who give birth (one in five moms), and it is considered to be the most common complication of childbirth. Postpartum psychosis, on the other hand, is incredibly rare and is thought to affect approximately one to two of every 1,000 women who deliver (approximately 0.01 percent). A 5 percent infanticide and suicide rate exists for those women who develop postpartum psychosis. The onset of postpartum psychosis is usually sudden and most often occurs within the first few weeks postpartum. The greatest known risk factors for developing PPP include a personal or family history of bipolar disorder or a previous psychotic episode. Symptoms of PPP are considered an emergency, and PPP requires immediate medical attention.

According to Postpartum Support International, some of the symptoms of postpartum psychosis include:

- Hallucinations (seeing things that are not there)
- Delusions and strange thoughts
- Hyperactivity
- Decreased need for or inability to sleep
- Paranoia and suspiciousness
- Rapid mood swings
- Difficulty communicating at times

Often in the case of PPP, family and friends will be the first to notice that something is going on for a mom with PPP that needs immediate attention. Often these moms will be "acting strangely" or seem totally unlike themselves. Moms with postpartum psychosis are often not in touch with reality, and so they may not acknowledge that they are in great trouble.

Because it is a biochemical issue, medication is required as part of the treatment. With this said, moms who develop postpartum psychosis do get better and go on to live happy and healthy lives after they recover.

Finally, many moms who walk into my office are afraid that they have PPP or are going to develop psychosis. Please remember that usually moms who develop PPP are not in touch with reality and are not aware that something is wrong. If you are seeking out help and are attuned to the fact that you are struggling, you are most likely not suffering from PPP. While postpartum depression and postpartum anxiety (especially postpartum OCD, which involves often obsessive and scary thoughts of harm coming to one's baby) can be hugely scary, unsettling, and intolerable for many moms, these challenges are very different from postpartum psychosis. Again, postpartum psychosis is incredibly rare.

Postpartum PTSD: Risk Factors and Symptoms

I have become especially interested in the phenomenon of postpartum post-traumatic stress disorder (PTSD). I live and work in a community where "natural" choices and attachment parenting are both respected and expected by many. Bradley Method childbirth education classes are common. Many local women chose to have a home birth or deliver with a midwife in the hospital. Breastfeeding is often nonnegotiable for new moms just beginning their journey, and non-medicated birth is the preferred option for a large number of women here.

While a culture of success exists (meaning that many women do end up with the births that they had hoped for), many common realities take many women off guard: the emergency C-sections; the "cascade of interventions" during childbirth that may start with induction; the common breastfeeding challenges; the delivery by an OB who was not the preferred choice; the reality of pain in childbirth; the loss of sense of control that can occur for many, many women, especially those who have a prior history of trauma or abuse; the premature baby or baby with medical issues who lands a family in the NICU; and infants lost during childbirth or shortly after. These things can happen, no matter how "prepared" or well-intentioned moms and medical providers are.

Often, I see these moms in my office weeks, months, and sometimes years after they experience a birth that was in some way "traumatic" for them. I put this word in quotes because we know by now that it is not the specifics of the birth events that can lead a mom to be traumatized, but her perception of these events. On paper, a birth might look "perfect" when, in reality, a mom may be walking away from her experience with some significant post-traumatic stress. Physicians, midwives, doulas, nurses, spouses, partners, and family members may assume that all is fine and dandy for a mom after she delivers a healthy newborn when, in reality, her perception is very, very different.

When looking at the probable "causes" of postpartum post-traumatic stress disorder, this is what we know may contribute to risk:

- **A perception of lack of caring:** Moms feel abandoned by providers or partners during their pregnancy or childbirth experience; moms do not feel reassured or supported during childbirth.
- **Poor communication:** Moms feel unheard during childbirth and feel that their perspectives around choices were not validated. Moms feel uninformed about choices being made to benefit her and her baby during childbirth.
- **Feelings of powerlessness:** Moms feel unprotected and under-supported by medical/birth staff. Moms feel that they had no control over the birth process.

- **A re-triggering of old trauma histories or fears:** Moms went into childbirth with intense fear and uncertainty that was not addressed.
- **A perception that a healthy baby was the only focus:** Moms feel that the attention was on the health and well-being of her baby while she went "unnoticed."

The reality is that postpartum PTSD is not that uncommon. Statistics vary, but the one that I have seen the most is a whopping 9 percent of women who deliver a baby will go on to develop symptoms of post-traumatic stress after birth. A study published in Birth: Issues in Perinatal Care broke these symptoms down into three categories.

- **Intrusion symptoms:** Repetitive re-experiencing of the birth trauma through flashbacks, nightmares, distressing recollections of the birth experience, and psychological distress following birth.
- **Avoidance symptoms:** Attempts to avoid reminders of the birth experience such as doctors' offices and hospitals, people associated with the birth experience (sometimes including the baby), and thoughts about the birth experience.
- **Increased arousal symptoms:** Difficulty sleeping, heightened anxiety, irritability, and concentration challenges.

Significant consequences exist for moms with postpartum PTSD if support isn't put into place. Moms who suffer from PTSD are less likely to have subsequent births (and are more likely to have an epidural or a scheduled C-section if/when they do); they are less likely to receive follow-up medical care; they are less likely to breastfeed (due to pain, feelings of violation, low milk supply, self-doubt and lack of confidence, and/or painful reminders of childbirth); they are more likely to have challenges bonding and attaching with their newborns (again, often due to triggering reminders of events); and they are more likely to experience conflict in their marriages/relationships and experience sexual dysfunction. Moms who suffer from postpartum PTSD are more likely to also suffer from depression.

We know that risk factors such as prenatal depression, a lack of social support, previous trauma histories, breastfeeding challenges, and physical challenges following childbirth can heighten a woman's reaction to trauma. But we also know that preventive measures such as well-established stress management strategies; "health-promoting behavior" such as healthy sleep, good nutrition, and exercise; and opportunities to debrief birth experiences can reduce a mom's risk for PTSD. In other words, with effort, some of these postpartum PTSD stories can be lessened.

Why is it important to know whether a mom has postpartum PTSD? Because in many cases, women are treated for their depression (remember, most women with PTSD will also be depressed), and their PTSD is not addressed. If a mom isn't asked the right questions and if she does not tell the whole story, she may be in treatment for a long time without gaining the desired relief. A mom with postpartum PTSD needs support in re-processing the experiences that led her there, in understanding why she developed the reaction that she did, and in understanding the role of old and new beliefs that may have led her to her reaction to her birth or that have been created due to her experience during childbirth. These women benefit greatly from having an opportunity to re-frame and better understand their birth experience for what it was—to them. For many women, specific work around trauma is necessary.

It is a great honor to be given access to a mom's story during birth, whether it was one that met her expectations or one that was upsetting and "traumatic." These stories are a woman's first experience with being a mom to a baby on the outside, and the ones that will often inform her earliest parts of motherhood. What was your birth story?

For additional support and information on postpartum PTSD, see the Resources section at the end of this book.

Post-Adoption Depression Syndrome (PADS)

Let's touch on another topic related to postpartum depression and anxiety: post-adoption depression syndrome (PADS). Today, many parents are adopting children, and it is important that we treat the inevitable challenges that come with this new role with the same importance that we do the challenges that come for postpartum women. Moms who adopt babies may not experience the potential struggle that accompanies hormonal shifts following birth, but they certainly do experience the same sleep deprivation, identity shifting, and adjustment challenges that every new mom faces. Often adoption brings additional challenges as well.

In an article in *The New York Times,* author Tara Parker-Pope touches on these challenges. Many new adoptive parents, she notes, have spent months or years in the process of adopting their child and, in doing so, work to prove that they will be exceptional parents. When their baby arrives, they—like every new parent—are faced with the realities that come with parenting and are often saddened or overwhelmed by the fact that they are not the "perfect" parents they portrayed themselves to be. This challenge of meeting unrealistic expectations is one contributing factor in the development of postpartum depression and anxiety, and it can often be the piece that is the hardest for new moms to accept. None of us are perfect. But just imagine what it would be like if you spent large amounts of time talking to others about the kind of "super parent" you will be, and then how disheartening it would be to realize, once your baby is home, that you can't possibly live up to this expectation. I suspect that many of us can relate to this situation.

In addition, many of these moms may have struggled through infertility treatments or the loss that comes with the realization that they are unable to conceive. While a new baby brings hope and excitement, significant sadness can come with the need to let go of the idea of carrying a biological baby of one's own.

So, if you have adopted a baby, please know that you are not alone in your struggles. For support and information related to PADS, its causes, and suggestions for how to deal with these challenges, visit adopting.org.

An Explanation of Suicidal Thinking in Plain Mama English

A new mom once asked me the following question:

What is considered a "suicidal" thought, ideation, or gesture? I remember being asked by my physician if I was having suicidal thoughts, and I honestly didn't know if I should say yes or no. I wasn't making plans in my head to kill myself when I was in the deepest throes of depression, but I was having weird fleeting thoughts about things like "what would it be like to throw myself down the stairs?" and "my family would be so much better off without me here because I cause them so much stress," etc. There were many days that I know I just kept holding on because my baby needed me and loved me and I couldn't bear the thought of leaving him. But was this considered being suicidal? I honestly still don't know. When you look up "suicidal thoughts" on medical websites, there's no plain mama English description on what this could be; it is focused on the emergent symptoms and description of planning and/or acting on these plans to try to kill yourself. I figure other moms out there may be just as clueless as I am, and it could be useful to have a plain mama description of this so we know if we should say yes or no to that scary question from our doctors.

It is a terrifying place to be when the thought of suicide or harming yourself comes into your head. Moms who suffer from postpartum depression do not always go to this place even though they may be suffering greatly. But those who do are usually dealt an additional level of uncertainty and fear: *Does this mean that I am really crazy? Will I be locked up for these thoughts that I am having? Will my baby be taken away? Will anyone even notice if I am no longer here?* Usually, for these moms, the thought of harm and/or suicide comes from one of two places: either the belief that her family will be better off without her or the feeling that she is in so much pain that she can't go on.

These thoughts can come in a wide variety of forms. Some moms are in such distress that they have fleeting thoughts of wanting to escape it all. Some moms have fleeting thoughts about putting themselves in harm's way. Other moms know that, despite their thoughts, they would never choose to follow through with these actions. Some moms wonder if they might follow through if things get bad enough. Other moms have a plan about what they would do to hurt themselves. And some moms have already made a commitment to do so.

So, as for the question above:

What, in "plain mama English," is suicidal thinking?

Technically speaking, a mom is having "suicidal thoughts" if and when she begins to think about hurting herself and/or ending her life. These thoughts are, indeed, red flags and a very necessary reason to seek out help. It is true that not every mom with postpartum depression having these thoughts will act them out, but any time that the thoughts occur, those of us in the field of postpartum depression treatment and mental health will pay attention and note that a mom is really deeply suffering.

In my practice, whenever a mom talks about having had thoughts like this, I put my "medication talk" in a whole new category. Medications are a very important part of treatment for moderate to severe cases of postpartum depression and are usually a relatively quick way to reduce symptoms. My preference for treatment that includes medication in these instances is NOT because I think these moms are "crazy" or "insane" or "unfit" to be moms, but rather because I know from their thoughts that they are suffering greatly, and I simply don't want them to have to struggle like that.

Clinically, a "suicide assessment" has to be done any time a mom (or any other individual) discloses that she is having thoughts of hurting herself or ending her life. When moms, like the one above, disclose these thoughts and then assure me that they have no intention of following through, I will make a verbal commitment with them that they will let me know if they do begin to think seriously about acting upon these thoughts or if these "thoughts" become "urges" (meaning that they are being drawn by an impulse to act upon their thoughts). If they are not doing so already, I will let them know that I think medication treatment is imperative. For moms who have a plan or who fear that they really may put themselves in harm's way, hospitalization is a necessary part of their treatment simply in order to get them immediate relief and to protect them.

Examples of Suicidal Thoughts

The Mayo Clinic lists the following as "warning signs" for suicidal thinking:

- Talking about suicide, including making such statements as "I'm going to kill myself," "I wish I were dead," or "I wish I hadn't been born."
- Getting the means to commit suicide, such as getting a gun or stock piling pills
- Withdrawing from social contact and wanting to be left alone
- Having mood swings, such as being emotionally high one day and deeply discouraged the next
- Being preoccupied with death, dying, or violence
- Feeling trapped or hopeless about a situation
- Increased use of alcohol or drugs
- Changing normal routine, including eating or sleeping patterns
- Doing risky or self-destructive things, such as using drugs or driving recklessly
- Giving away belongings or getting affairs in order
- Saying goodbye to people as if they won't be seen again
- Developing personality changes, such as becoming very outgoing after being shy

Any time a mom with postpartum depression is struggling with the above symptoms, it is absolutely imperative for her to reach out for appropriate support, even if it is hard to do so. In fact, acknowledging suicidal thoughts, answering "yes" when asked if you're having suicidal thoughts, and being honest with yourself and others is usually the hardest part. But please, please know that you do not need to suffer in this way. Even if you have gotten very used to doing so. You owe it to yourself to live your life without these (even fleeting) thoughts or fears. And your babies and families do need you.

Winter Blues: What You Need to Know about Seasonal Affective Disorder and PPD

Winter. It can be a tough time for all of us. The days get shorter and colder, the weather is often chaotic, the roads are sometimes dangerous, and the gas bills go up. Fresh fruits and vegetables can be harder to find and usually become more expensive in these long months. Runny noses abound, and the flu seems to be around every corner. The air gets drier, our skin cracks, and we often are not drinking enough water. Children tend to go stir-crazy when their playtime outdoors is limited. And, if we do attempt to get those little ones outside, our efforts at managing struggling kiddos into appropriate layers can feel for naught when red-cheeked toddlers decide that they are cold and wet after only a few minutes of play.

Winter tends to be a time when our neighbors are rarely seen, when communities are harder to access, and when we find ourselves spending more time at home. We tend to lose our patience more often. We tend to have a harder time concentrating. We often have less energy. We feel less creative. We might, even, suffer from a bit of seasonal affective disorder (SAD).

While winters are mild and seasons nonexistent in many parts of the world, daylight levels lessen in the winter months unless you are living on or very near to the equator. Less daylight can lead to an increase in melatonin production that, in turn, can increase feelings of lethargy. Sunlight is also a major source of the vitamin D that we receive, and decreases in vitamin D have been associated with symptoms of depression and anxiety.

It is highly common for people to spend more time sleeping in the winter months, for daytime fatigue to set in, appetites to increase, and moods to dampen. Think hibernation. Often, as the days become shorter and darker and the weather less accommodating, many of us find ourselves wishing that we could crawl into a cave and hibernate with the bears.

If you are struggling with postpartum depression or another postpartum mood and anxiety disorder, winters can feel long and intolerable.

I see the effects of the overlap between postpartum depression and SAD—or what I will call "winter blues"—in my private psychotherapy practice. The phone rings more and the referrals come in more frequently. This makes sense, doesn't it? We know that the keys to a healthy postpartum experience and often the important pieces of a mom's recovery involve community support, exercise, healthy nutrition and adequate water intake, fresh air and breath, and rest.

Consider this image:

A new mom lives in an area where the winter is long and dark and cold. She has recently given birth, and her partner has returned to work. Biologically, she is craving more sleep and winter fatigue has set in, but her baby is fussy and she is unable to get the rest that she so greatly needs and desires. The roads are slippery, and her increasing anxiety is making it feel nearly impossible to venture out to see friends, or get to that moms' group she has been considering, or try the day care at the gym so that she can finally get some exercise. It is too cold and wet to walk outside as she worries about her baby in such weather. Her refrigerator is empty, and although she knows that healthy food and fresh vegetables might make a difference in how she feels, she doubts that she will ever manage the shopping that is required for this. Her skin is dry and she knows that she would benefit from drinking more water, but the cold weather makes it less desirable to do so. Her lack of perspective is making these months feel like forever, and she feels entirely unable to imagine that these long months will ever end.

The National Institutes of Health (NIH) lists the following as symptoms of seasonal affective disorder (SAD).

- Increased appetite with weight gain (weight loss is more common with other forms of depression)
- Increased sleep and daytime sleepiness (too little sleep is more common with other forms of depression)
- Less energy and ability to concentrate in the afternoon
- Loss of interest in work or other activities
- Slow, sluggish, lethargic movement
- Social withdrawal
- Unhappiness and irritability

For women who are caring for newborns during these months, symptoms of PPD and SAD can combine to create a perfect storm of distress.

If you are a new mother living in a part of the world where you are experiencing winter and reduced sunlight, there are a few things that you can do that might help. While we have plenty of evidence to suggest that seasonal affective disorder may heighten the feelings of depression for mothers, we also know that these risks can be limited by the following:

~ Get outside every day. If it's freezing out, bundle up! 15-30 minutes of sunlight a day (without the use of sunglasses if you are out early: I note morning) will help.

~ Move your body. During the winter months when our access to sunlight lessons, we want to increase other lifestyle choices that lead to good health. Exercise and move meant is one of those things. Take a walk outside for those 15-30 minutes of sun exposure, dance in your kitchen, do jumping jacks. It doesn't really matter. Just move.

~ Light-box therapy can be useful for those folks who are extra susceptible to Seasonal Affective Disorders (SAD) and who live in parts of the world where the sun does not shine in the winter. Talk to your health professional about this option.

If you are able to continue to care for yourself in the winter months by allowing yourself to slow down while also accessing vitamin D and exercise where you can, you will likely find that you feel less impacts of the winter blues.

Can You Get Postpartum Depression *after* the First Year?

I often receive calls from moms whose kiddos are past the one-year mark. Sometimes I even receive calls from moms whose kiddos are as "old" as three. These moms always start the same way: "My son/daughter is almost (one, two, three years old), and so I know that I don't have postpartum depression. But I am really unhappy and think that I need help. I know that your specialty is PPD, so can I still make an appointment to see you?"

While I can't make a blanket statement about each and every woman who calls me, more times than not these women—one, two, or three years past the birth of their little ones—are struggling with a form of maternal distress that dates back, in one way or another, to their pregnancy, postpartum, or even before. While these moms wouldn't technically have postpartum depression any longer, they are often struggling with what I will call here *continued postpartum distress* that was never adequately supported when they first noticed symptoms.

When we use the terms *prenatal/antenatal* and *postpartum depression*, we are really simply talking about an episode of depression or anxiety that occurs sometime during pregnancy or the first year postpartum. We believe that early symptoms, whether mild or severe, are caused by hormonal shifts during pregnancy or following delivery, physiological stressors like sleep deprivation and nutrient depletion, psychological strain including thought patterns that are likely to cause distress (such as "should" statements, perfectionist thinking, black or white thinking, and catastrophic thoughts), and/or other environmental stressors such as trauma, relationship conflict, or changes in finances, employment, or residence.

A postpartum episode of depression or anxiety can be triggered by one or more of the above. While they aren't aware of this when they first call, most of these moms can trace their initial symptoms back to the earliest moments of motherhood. On the phone before they come in for a full assessment session, these moms will say things like, *"But I was fine after I had my baby, and I didn't start feeling bad until later.*

However, any one or more of the following are usually what we discover when we are together in my office.

1. This mom has a long personal or family history of diagnosed or undiagnosed depression, anxiety, or mental illness.
2. The pregnancy wasn't planned, and this mom wasn't certain that she wanted to be pregnant, although she never disclosed this with anyone.
3. This mom had a difficult delivery that was never fully processed after her birth.

4. This mom had significant breastfeeding challenges that she struggled with silently.
5. This mom describes her early postpartum months as "foggy" and notes that she actually doesn't remember enjoying them.
6. This mom had always hoped for a boy/girl, but gave birth to the other. While she loves her kiddo fiercely, she has never quite managed the loss she feels around not giving birth to the gender that she had dreamed of. Or perhaps this mom has always worried about her attachment to her child.
7. This mom experienced a move, the death of a loved one, financial loss, or relationship conflict around the time of her birth, and these environmental stressors were pushed aside because she felt she "should" be happy once her baby was born.
8. This mom had an early childhood trauma or serious family of origin conflict, and she notes that emotions around these issues resurfaced shortly after she gave birth.
9. This mom felt unsupported in the months after she gave birth and felt that she "had to do it all on her own."
10. This mom's baby did not sleep through the night until many months or years after he/she was born.
11. This mom has not wanted anyone other than herself or her partner to care for her baby, and so she has not taken more than a very short period of time away from her baby since he/she was born.
12. This mom became pregnant after months or years of fertility treatments; she used donor eggs to become pregnant; she had her baby through a surrogate; or she adopted her baby, and once becoming a mom she pushed all of her emotions around her efforts to become a mama aside.
13. This mom is tired. Unrelentingly, frustratingly, understandably, deeply tired.

While the beginning of motherhood can feel exciting (perhaps sometimes even euphoric) for many women, symptoms of depression and anxiety can develop or increase over such a subtle period of time that moms do not necessarily acknowledge that they are depressed or anxious until well into or past that first postpartum year. Often, stress can be cumulative. Months of inadequate sleep, poor nutrition, relationship conflict, and hidden emotional strain can take their toll on a brain.

Think of a minor running injury. While on a jog, you trip and feel a slight pinch in your knee. You keep running and barely notice it. But each time you get back out to go for a jog, your knee becomes more and more strained (yet not painful enough to keep you off your feet). Suddenly one day while running months later, your knee gives out.

It has had enough. Your brain can do the same.

Why is all of this important? Too often, women assume that they have found themselves in a life that is just characterized by suffering, and they assume that since they don't have postpartum depression, it is silly or unnecessary to reach out for support. And so they keep on trekking while each day feeling overwhelmed, anxious, and farther from the woman whom they know themselves to be.

We talk so much about postpartum mood and anxiety disorders and not enough about maternal distress, and I fear that many women tell themselves that they have missed the window of diagnosis or validity for their struggle.

While being a mother is wonderful, it is also complicated. Let's make room for both, no matter how far into the journey of motherhood you are.

Childbirth Outcomes and Postpartum Depression: Are They Linked?

Oh, the pressure around childbirth! Do we try for a natural, unmedicated birth, or do we choose an epidural to relieve our pain when delivering our little ones? Do we hire a doula to support us through our childbirth journey, or do we rely on our doctor and nurses to support us throughout? Do we choose to give birth in the comfort of our home with a trained home birth midwife, or do we plan to labor and deliver in a hospital surrounded by doctors and the option for pain medication? Do we choose to attempt a VBAC or plan a second C-section? Do we lean toward waiting for natural contractions to begin, or do we get induced and, with that, have a clear idea of when that little face will enter this world? Do we go forward toward childbirth with a birth plan, or do we enter the experience with an ease and flexibility about what the ultimate experience entails? These decisions can be endless, and I think it is fair to say that expectation, judgment, and pressures come at us from every direction as we muddle through this laundry list of "choices."

The woman and mother in me believe strongly that we should have a say in the process that is called birth. I believe that each woman should have the right to choose her care provider, what positions she wants to labor in, and whether or not to receive pain relief. Each one of us is, ultimately, the best judge of what our body needs under best-case scenarios. However, the clinician in me also knows that sometimes deep hopes and expectations can lead to emotional challenges postpartum if and when they are not met as desired. And the research buff, experienced therapist, and perinatal mood disorder specialist in me knows that it is actually not the specifics of one's birth that can lead to a postpartum mood disorder like postpartum depression, anxiety, or postpartum PTSD, but a mom's perceptions of those experiences.

Let me explain with some examples:

I am talking about the mom whose birth, on paper, was "perfect." She gave birth in a hospital with a nurse midwife. Her labor was moderate in length, and she delivered vaginally with no medication for pain relief. Her baby was born with an Apgar score of nine. Her husband was encouraging of her throughout. And, still, this mom arrived in my office several weeks later in deep despair. In her memory, her birth was "traumatic." She remembers intense pain and little relief from this, and while her husband and midwife had cheered her on because they "knew" that she had wanted to give birth naturally, what she remembers wanting most desperately was for it all to just stop. She cried when recalling that she felt unheard, torn apart, and vulnerable. She was terrified throughout her birth process, and despite the loving people around her, she felt very much alone. Because it had all gone as planned, this mom felt ashamed for her despair and guilty for "not being happy" about all of it. She had, until coming to my office, not talked to anyone about how she felt.

I am talking about the mom who wanted desperately to give birth "naturally," but who, after 30 hours of labor and six hours of pushing, was rushed into the operating room for an emergency C-section. A nurse held her hand all the way down the hall and explained to her what was happening. She remembers her OB, masked and ready for surgery, talking to her over the curtain as he explained his process in removing her son from her body. She remembers seeing her son whisked away after being born and being left, only momentarily, until a second nurse whom she had never met came and sat with her and described her baby in detail until her partner returned. When asked about her birth experience, this mom smiled and became tearful with pride. "It was as it was meant to be," she said. "My baby and I were surrounded by people who cared about us, and I could not have asked for anything more."

I am talking about the mom who is terrified of pain and who, leading up to her birth, knew that she wanted an epidural at the moment her contractions began. Her friends all discouraged her from this as most of them had given birth naturally without intervention, but this mom knew what was best for her and remained committed to this. Her epidural was followed by the typical cascade of interventions: Pitocin, heart monitor, and an ultimate vacuum delivery. She gave birth to a beautiful baby girl, with an OB whom she had never met, and with nurses whom she never got to know because of a shift change during her labor. "It was amazing," this mom says of her birth. "It was all that I hoped and expected."

Numerous opinions, camps of thought, and differing ideas exist about what it means to give birth. So many, in fact, that it is unrealistic and unfair to assume that any of us know what the "right way to give birth" is. What truly matters most in the connection between birth experience and whether or not a mom develops postpartum depression, postpartum PTSD, or any other mood disorder is whether or not she felt heard, seen, and supported, and whether or not that mom had the chance to process her experience and talk about what it means to her, both empowering and difficult. Truly. Even a mom who is disappointed by the loss of expectation around a hoped childbirth may not develop symptoms of depression or anxiety if she is given the chance to discuss and mourn her losses.

Every woman should have the chance to think about what she would like, ideally, and have the opportunity to express this to her care providers and her support people. One OB with whom I work closely here in Boulder (and whom I trust, admire, and respect deeply) speaks openly about how, if a mom does not express a desire to give birth without intervention, she will assume that an epidural and Pitocin will be part of the equation. And if a mom does not reject this, she will push on. Because, yes, in Western medicine this seems to be the culture these days. And so, I imagine that because of similar situations across the globe, we are led to believe that OBs don't care what a mom wants and that a mom really has to *fight* for the kind of birth that she desires.

And fighting is draining. And heart-wrenching. And leaves us feeling angry and let down and vulnerable even if we end up with what we want.

So, write your birth plan if that's something you'd like to do. Interview providers and find someone to work with who, ideally, supports your ultimate goals in childbirth if/whenever possible. If you are working with an OB in a practice with rotating providers, make sure that you meet each one and spread your hopes around so those doctors know who you are and what your ultimate wishes are in delivery care. Talk to your partner, your doula if you have one, and your doctor or midwife about your hopes and fears around childbirth and make sure that they know what kind of emotional support you desire. If you plan on delivering in a hospital, request a nurse who has experience supporting moms through natural childbirth if this is a goal (yes, you *can* request this). You can most certainly do your part ahead of time to set yourself up for the most supported experience possible.

Of course, know that it doesn't always go as planned. Know that many times your wishes won't be granted and your goals won't be met because birth tends to happen the way it happens both because of and despite our positive thinking, hard work, and determination. Sometimes we are pleasantly surprised, but often we find that our expectations result in a bit of loss. If this is you, please seek out support ASAP: from your partner, family members, friends, doula, doctor, or therapist ... wherever you can!

Our birth experiences tend to determine the lens from which we look into early motherhood, and if it doesn't feel right—if this lens is dusted with anger, disappointment, sadness, loss, or fear—you might be at a higher risk for developing postpartum depression, anxiety, or PTSD. The sooner you get support around this, the sooner you will be able to look toward being a mom with clarity and understanding.

Can PPD Be Prevented?

I am asked this question a lot. Experts believe that because there is no definite way of knowing how a woman's body will respond to childbirth, we cannot claim any specific prevention. However, I do believe that a woman and her family can do quite a bit during pregnancy and after birth that will lessen her chances of a postpartum mood and anxiety disorder like postpartum depression, or that may, at least, play a role in the reduction of symptoms.

So, let's go through them, shall we? Many people cringe at the idea of guarantees, but I might take a bit of a risk here and say that I most certainly can guarantee that if you focus on the things below, you will be reducing your risk of developing postpartum depression or anxiety. Reducing risk is an act of prevention. If you are already struggling? These things will help. Promise.

1. Nourishment

Nutrition and Protein: Recent research has shown significant correlation between nutrient depletion and symptoms of postpartum depression and anxiety. A pregnant or new mom's body will donate whatever nutrients are necessary to her baby, often at the cost of her own reserves. And growing a baby, childbirth, and breastfeeding all demand larger amounts of energy and nutrition than usual. It is easy to get depleted during these times. So, stockpile! If you are not already taking one, find a good prenatal vitamin that your tummy can tolerate (and if you have already delivered and have gone off your prenatal vitamin, go back on!). Consider adding an omega-3 supplement if your prenatal doesn't already include this. Omega-3 fatty acids are not only hugely important for your baby's brain development, but they have also been shown to aid in symptoms of depression and anxiety.

Our brains need healthy nutrition and protein to function adequately. In fact, the "feel good hormone" serotonin is not naturally occurring in our bodies, and therefore it requires important building blocks (amino acids/tryptophan) that come from the food we eat. A well-balanced diet with protein at every meal is required for optimal emotional well-being. Vegetarians and vegans will need to intentionally include plenty of eggs (for non-vegans) legumes, nuts, seeds, soy proteins and grains.

Water: Research suggests a connection between dehydration and anxiety. Moms who are pregnant, who deliver babies, and who breastfeed are at an especially high risk for problems associated with inadequate water intake. Drink up.

Pampering and self-care: Yes, this is even important once your baby comes. Please remember that self-care is NOT selfish and that your baby needs you to be well. Nourish yourself all that you can with breaks when needed, baths, time with friends, and whatever else your brain and body need to feel grounded. Your baby needs you to be mentally and physically healthy when that baby is on the outside, too, so don't stop taking care of yourself. Ever.

2. Rest

Adequate sleep: While having a newborn certainly does make it difficult to get the same quality/quantity of sleep you got before you were a mama, sleep deprivation should be monitored. Studies have shown that quality of sleep is a higher predictor for postpartum depression and anxiety than the temperament of one's baby, meaning a mom with a difficult baby who gets "enough" sleep is less likely to become depressed/anxious than a mom with an "easy baby" who is sleep-deprived, and so getting enough sleep cannot be emphasized enough. For women with a prior mental health concern (especially bipolar disorder), adequate sleep can make the difference in preventing relapse. Consider aiming for at least one block of four hours of uninterrupted sleep a night (at a minimum). This block of sleep can occur at any point. (Hint: Most healthy babies will give you a chunk of sleep sometime between 7p.m. and midnight.)

3. Exercise and Movement

Stay as active as possible: Women who get some form of mild to moderate exercise each day are generally less likely to become depressed or anxious than those who do not. This does not mean that you must go to the gym. Or run a marathon. Or even get out to attend a yoga class. What we are referring to here is "movement and activity," as this helps the increase of endorphins and the decrease of stress hormones like cortisol. While it is completely normal and expected that your "regular" exercise routine will change during pregnancy (due to increased fatigue, movement difficulty, aches and pains, or doctor's orders), some form of mild to moderate physical activity is important whenever possible. By the way, you will have the energy to return to a vigorous exercise habit again once you have healed from childbirth if this is important to you! Research has shown that women who continue mild to moderate physical activity during pregnancy have a quicker physical recovery postpartum and tend to suffer less from depression and/or anxiety. So, go for walks, take the stairs, go for a swim, or stretch at home, unless otherwise instructed by your health care provider. While some women will be able to continue to run, bike, and do other heartier exercise into their last trimester, this tends to be rare. The key is to listen to your body. When it tells you to stop or slow down, it's time to listen.

4. Support

Create your village: Did you know that our nervous systems respond to connection? In moments of connection with others, our parasympathetic nervous systems turn on and our heart rates slow, our breath deepens, and our bodies relax. It makes sense, then, that inadequate social support is one of the leading factors in developing depression or anxiety postpartum. Along with the calming impact to our nervous systems, community and connection with others allow for validation and emotional and logistical support.

The saying "It takes a village to raise a child" should apply to all of us. Yet for some reason, many women in our society assume that we should be able to "do it all" on our own, and this often leaves us feeling depleted and isolated. So, while it may feel uncomfortable to reach out initially, doing so while still pregnant will ease things up once that babe arrives (and people actually really do love to help!). Sign people up long before your due date, if possible. Some ideas for support? Identify people you trust whom you can rely on for emotional support and encouragement; enlist people you can rely on to give you breaks on a regular basis; ask someone to organize a food drop-off for the weeks after your baby arrives. Your own self-nourishment is imperative in motherhood—having someone hold or feed your baby so that you can shower, nap, go for a walk, go to a yoga class, see friends, get a massage, and whatever else feels good is as important for your baby as it is for you!

If you are at risk for PPD, consider finding a psychotherapist whom you trust now: I can't tell you how many calls I get from moms who have been suffering for months before they finally reach out. If these moms, many of whom were in the high-risk category for a perinatal mood and anxiety disorder before becoming pregnant, had reached out for support during their pregnancy, months of needless suffering may have been prevented. Working with a therapist to prepare for the emotional journey into motherhood could be all that you need to glide gracefully through this transition.

If you are taking medication for depression and/or anxiety, remain on it unless you are under the supervision of a health care provider trained in PPD: Many women make the mistake of taking themselves off their meds without the guidance of their MD, midwife, or therapist. Women who struggle with depression and/or anxiety during pregnancy are 50 percent more likely to develop PPD, and so preparing accordingly is imperative. Many medications have been shown to be safe to take while pregnant and also while breastfeeding, and the risks of untreated depression and anxiety outweigh the risks of these meds to your unborn or nursing babe. If you have questions or concerns about this, talk to your health care provider.

Find a moms' group: Again, the power of community support cannot be understated. Mom and baby groups provide a network of other moms who are going through the same things that you are; a space to share excitement, challenges, and strategies; and a reason to get dressed and out into the world each week. So do a little research now and see what your options are!

Talk to others: It is so easy to feel enveloped in your sense of being overwhelmed in the first few weeks and months of motherhood. At some point, just about everyone gets nervous about the changing colors of poop, the quantities of spit-up, and the baby who just won't seem to sleep. Yet, when you put your concerns and anxieties out into the world, you will realize that just about every new mom is feeling the same way. So share your experiences—the good, the bad, *and* the ugly.

5. Understanding and Awareness

Get curious about you: Women who know their risk for a postpartum mood and anxiety disorder are less likely to be hit unexpectedly with an episode of depression and anxiety and are more likely to put preventive measures into place. Understanding how your brain works, what your vulnerabilities and triggers are, and what you need most to feel well can make all the difference in your postpartum recovery. Please make sure that your expectations of yourself are realistic!

Get curious about your partner: It has also been shown that couples who discuss their parenting hopes, expectations, fears, and roles prior to the birth of a baby are much more equipped to support each other along the way. The first postpartum year is a tough one for couples, and the more you communicate before your baby arrives, the more equipped you will be to manage the challenges. Learn what each of you wants out of being a parent and what type of parent you each dream of becoming. Inform each other now about what types of support are important to you. Plan ahead for how to give each other breaks, especially around nighttime and sleep. And go into this wonderfully challenging adventure with realistic ideas and patience for each other's process.

Be realistic! Those myths and unrealistic expectations about motherhood are dangerous. While becoming a mother is, truly, one of the most rewarding and wonderful opportunities imaginable, it comes complete with frustration, overwhelm, uncertainty, fear, and heartache. Those magazine images of size 6 bodies weeks after birth and images of wonderfully content (all the time) women breastfeeding their happy babies in spotless homes are simply not realistic. Motherhood is messy and unpredictable. Breastfeeding is initially challenging for most. You might wonder why you wanted to be a mother so badly and look, momentarily, for a way out. Yet, despite the momentary daydreams of faraway places, the dishes that pile up, the pj's at noon, and the probability of tears, you are still being a great mom who is doing her best. It is important to realize how absolutely normal it is to feel unsettled in your role for a while. Almost every mom does!

Expect some old stuff to resurface: It is amazing how much old stuff can come creeping back to the surface after a baby is born ... no matter how long you have worked on it in the past or how "over it" you feel. While it doesn't happen for everyone, most moms will suddenly find that old patterns with family members (especially parents) creep back in unexpectedly. If this happens, be kind to yourself. Talking to your partner, a close friend, and/or a therapist can help you get through this challenge more quickly.

6. Stress Management

Becoming a mother and having a new baby are simply stressful at times. There is no way around this one, and it is entirely normal to have moments of anxiety, irritability, and sadness along the way. What is important, however, is that moms have some tools for managing the emotions that come up when times get hard. Moms who have access to stress reduction strategies are less likely to become depressed and anxious than moms who do not.

Breath: When we are stressed or anxious, most of us are not breathing adequately. When we breathe with our full lung capacity—all the way to the bottom of our lungs (diaphragmatic breathing)—we give our brains the amount of fresh oxygen they need to function efficiently. Breathing effectively can literally change our bodies' physiological response to stress.

Deep relaxation strategies: When we are stressed and anxious, we often forget what it feels like to be relaxed. Reminding your body that this is possible is important. There are a number of tools you can use:

- **Progressive relaxation:** In a lying-down or comfortable position, tense and relax each part of your body either from head to toe or from toe to head. Notice what it feels like to be tense (in your toes, foot, calf, and onward) and then what it feels like to be completely relaxed. When you have gone through each body part in succession, tense and then release your entire body at once. This is often a great tool when you're having a hard time falling asleep.
- **Visualization:** Think of or make up a place that gives you the sense of total relaxation. This can be some place that you have been before or a place that you have dreamed of. Close your eyes and see if you can bring yourself there: What do you see? What do you hear? What do you feel? What do you smell? What do you taste? While you do this, remember to practice your deep breathing. Notice, sense, and feel how your body reacts to this place. When you have reached a sense of calm and well-being, open your eyes. You can return to this place any time that you need it.
- **Grounding exercises:** Often, anxiety (including panic) includes a sense of being not grounded, floating, or ruminating about the past or future. Reminding yourself to be in the moment can decrease the symptoms that accompany the inability to be present. To do this, notice, and say out loud, where you are in the moment. What do you see? What do you hear? What do you feel? What do you taste? What do you smell? This exercise

can take as much or as little time as you have. The goal is to bring yourself back to the moment.

Please remember, folks, even women who do the above can suffer through a postpartum mood and anxiety disorder like PPD. Sometimes a mom's symptoms will get in the way of accessing these strategies, and sometimes a mom's depression and/or anxiety will be at a level that is distressing no matter what she "does." Doing everything possible to take care of yourself isn't a guarantee that you won't have PPD. At the same time, it can feel incredibly empowering to do what you can to care for yourself. And if you are a mom who is recovering from postpartum depression, know that the above strategies may help you to thrive, one baby step at a time.

When Conceiving Isn't Easy

Let's not get too far ahead of ourselves without both honoring and shining a light on the moms out there who have struggled to get pregnant- who have taken a number of rides on that rollercoaster called *fertility treatments*, who have hoped and prayed and bargained and begged to finally conceive.

The fertility journey is no joke. And data informs us that 19% of us will struggle with infertility issues. That's a lot of hope and heartbreak.

For those of you who have been down this road, we see you. If you have become pregnant and carried a baby to term after these trials and tribulations, you are likely both relieved and grateful and also exhausted and grief stricken. The losses for moms who go through the fertility journey are often subtle and hidden from view, and so many mothers feel very alone in this journey. The failed IV transfers, the unexpected periods, and the unhealthy embryos are all major losses for moms. The successful transfers and the ultimate healthy pregnancies that happen are blessings and worthy of celebration of course, but amidst this joy is very often a quiet pain lingering in the background.

Moms who get pregnant after assisted reproduction efforts are at a higher risk for developing a PMAD like postpartum depression for a number of reasons:

They enter pregnancy with an exhausted hormonal system already.

There may not be adequate space to grieve the losses through the fertility journey, and so those harder and more complicated feelings linger.

The people around these moms communicate the blessings in all-or-nothing ways *"It's all ok now! You finally got your baby!"* or, *"It was all worth it, right?"* are common responses to a new mom who has worked hard to conceive. And it's not that these things aren't true- they certainly often are. But these statements neglect the other complicated parts of the journey.

For many families, fertility treatments are a financial strain. So, once that baby arrives, the stress associated with becoming parents lingers.

So, if this is you, be kind to yourself. Find other moms out there who have gone through that journey too (there are many). Seek out a safe space to share all of your feelings- especially the ones that feel more hidden from view. Every single emotion you are having makes sense.

That baby is very lucky to have you. You have worked hard to bring him/her into this world. Now it's time to take care of you.

II. BIOLOGICAL HEALTH:
Your Brain & Your Body

From First Bleed to Last: The Progression of Reproductive Mental Health

It's interesting (and perhaps a little startling) to consider that from the moment an adolescent girl has her first period, she enters the world of *motherhood*. A first period doesn't just mean logistical frustration and uncertainty, it also means that her body is capable of carrying a *baby*. It is at this point that girls are taught (or learn on their own) about the risks of pregnancy, and are either shamed or (hopefully) empowered toward self-protection, making sure that they do not become pregnant before they are ready. A girl's hormones are in high gear during this time of body development and physiological instability, and we see her moods change. She might be more tearful, more anxious, and more vulnerable to stress. **This is a time when mental health diagnoses like depression and anxiety are often first called to attention.** Not only are these female teenaged brains adjusting to hormone fluctuations, but they are also developing in maturity to allow for more self-awareness and big-picture thinking. Throughout her teenage years and early adulthood, she may ponder the question *"Do I want to have children?"* Throughout this season of her development, she might find herself excited or daunted (or both!) by the possibility. Without a doubt, she will feel something when considering the question (even if the feeling looks like numbness or "*I-don't-know-ness*" or resistance to the thought). **This first bleed is when the possibility of becoming a mother first becomes real.**

I was a girl myself, and now I have two daughters, one, 14, who has bled already and one, 12, who is on the brink, as noted by the mood swings, fatigue, and body development. As a maternal mental health specialist, it is fascinating to watch.

Once these girls become young women and are in some kind of a groove of early adulthood and pregnancy protection, they might stop considering motherhood so explicitly for a while. It is a time of rest for the female brain. The waves show up once a month as these young women navigate the often-rough waters of pre- and post-menstrual cycles, but once they are outside of adolescence and first periods, this hormonal-related mental health crisis of sorts often begins to settle.

Rest while you can, female brain.

Because then, for those who choose to become mothers or who become mothers unexpectedly, conception, pregnancy, and postpartum will arrive at some point. Hormones like estrogen and progestogen rev their motors again and come out in full force at the moment of conception. Periods stop, but reproductive systems start their jobs as best they can to orient everything in the female body toward producing a healthy baby. Once again, the waves of emotional instability roll in with inevitable force. Periods stop, temporarily, and emotions become more vibrant. Within 24 hours of childbirth, a mother's levels of estrogen and progesterone can drop to below 200 times their pre-pregnancy levels. The female brain tries to rebound from this shift in chemistry, but it often cannot. **One in five new moms will struggle with a postpartum mood and anxiety disorder like postpartum depression as, once again, the reproductive cycle has stirred up some chaos in mood.** This is the second time in a female's life when rates of depression and anxiety increase in the population.

Ideally, mothers get support and treatment if they need it. As her period starts again sometime after childbirth, a woman is likely to feel the now-familiar shifts in brain chemistry and mood with an unexpected force, as the monthly roller-coaster ride starts up again. Her cycle will find its groove again, but this takes some time. She will find some relief in predictability and rhythm, but if she has another baby, the cycle of periods stopping and hormones increasing will take her on another journey through increased vulnerability—it is unavoidable. Hopefully, by this point, a mother understands her body's response to pregnancy, and has established some techniques for coping and accessing support. Ideally, she feels more ready to tolerate the chaos of hormone-related mental health challenges.

Ahhh ... but perhaps not for long. Women are having babies later in life than they used to. In fact, the average age of a first-time mother in Boulder, where I live, is 37.

Cue up perimenopause. The reproductive mental health performance continues.

In come "irregular periods," hot flashes, dryness in every place possible, and,

yes, mood instability all over again. The female body is preparing to let go of its job in reproduction, and so the hormones required for this incredible feat are disappearing. Sometimes slowly, and sometimes with a force that shakes the ground like never before. I am just starting this journey toward menopause myself. (Menopause, if you didn't know, is actually the one day in which you hit 12 months with no period. Perimenopause can last for years.) I am putting my seat belt on as we speak. As someone who suffered from a postpartum anxiety disorder, I am at risk of heightened mental health challenge during this final stage of reproductive activity in my body. The self-caretaking I do at this time will help to soften the blow to my mental health as I endure this final season of change.

Menopause may feel like a logistical relief for many women, but it is also a shift in season of life and there is inevitably a letting go that occurs. The reproductive system has done its job. Its performance is over. The curtain goes down on the possibility of becoming pregnant and carrying a child. With all loss, there is a period of grief, and many women will feel grief as they face the idea of motherhood again. This time with a farewell.

From first bleed to last, a female brain is at the mercy of the hormones that seem to come out of nowhere and then disappear again. Of course, they are not gone altogether, but their job in the making of a mother is done.

Brain Science and Postpartum Anxiety

I went to a phenomenal talk once in which Kristen Race, PhD, talked about the science behind stress in kids. While her talk was aimed at understanding children's responses to stress, much of what she discussed is absolutely appropriate—and fitting—when trying to understand some of the science behind anxiety in the postpartum period.

So much research has been conducted recently on the neurobiology of psychology, the neurobiology of attachment, and other related fields of study. We know that much of the way we behave, react, and interact with the world is due to neural pathways (or well-paved roads) in our brains that have been formed through repetitive events and experience. Unconsciously, much of our behavior is due to our procedural memory—ways of interacting and reacting to the world that come instinctively due to what we have experienced or what we "know." This "procedural memory" is implicit and often presents itself at times when we are "triggered" by something. For example, if you were raised in a household where it was not okay to cry or show emotion, you may become extremely uncomfortable, anxious, or overwhelmed when your own baby cries, because your "procedural memory" is triggered, and you make the connection (unconsciously) that crying is scary and not okay.

Are you still with me?

The next piece is what I brought with me from Kristen's talk and the part I find most fascinating. Postpartum depression (PPD) and other perinatal mood disorders are known to be what we call a bio, psycho, and social issue, meaning that they are caused by disruptions in a woman's biology (hormone fluctuations, personal or family history of mental illness, sleep deprivation, nutritional depletion, etc.), psychology (thought patterns, identity, etc.), and social network (social support, family of origin issues, etc.). Any woman who gives birth to a baby is at risk of developing PPD or postpartum anxiety (PPA) due to the simple fact that her hormones are in flux (please note that we also know that adoptive moms, non-birth mothers,_and dads can also suffer from perinatal mood and anxiety disorders, or PMADS, even though they have not given birth). With additional stressors in her life, she may be even more vulnerable during the postpartum period.

In Kristin's talk, she mapped out the ways that children's brains react to stress: When kids do not have enough structure, when they lack routine or do not know what to expect next, and when they feel a lack of control, they function out of the amygdala (or the brain stem), which is responsible for "fight or flight" reactions. In other words, they tend to be highly anxious, irritable, and agitated. The part of the brain responsible for reason, problem-solving, and clear thought is the prefrontal cortex—and this part of the brain functions most efficiently when there is consistency, routine, structure, and expectation.

Get where I'm going with this?

New moms in the first several weeks and months after bringing a baby home are existing in a new reality that usually involves a lack of routine, lack of structure, lack of control, and an inability to have any idea of what to expect next. Babies cry and we don't know why. Minutes turn into hours turn into days and mom still hasn't made it past her front porch (unless she finally got to the grocery store, which can feel like climbing Mount Everest). It feels impossible to plan much of anything, and so regular routines seem like a thing of the past. For many new moms, this first period of motherhood feels just plain chaotic.

What part of the brain takes over when in these situations? The amygdala, responsible for "fight or flight" reactions, for emotion, for anxiety, and for agitation. When this part of the brain is on fire, it is literally impossible to expect to think rationally and problem solve. When we are in this place, we must work hard to wake up the prefrontal cortex, which is responsible for this type of clear-headedness. In other words, during the postpartum period when routine, structure, and expectation fly out the window, it is scientifically probable that a mom will be anxious because of the way her brain is working with all the unknowns.

I talked to Kristin about this to make sure I was making a clear connection, and she confirmed my assumptions about this with respect to new moms. However, I am not a neuroscientist nor do I intend to come up with a new theory on what causes postpartum anxiety. Sometimes it's just helpful to be reminded that the intense emotions and struggles that moms face are biological and scientific in nature and not because moms are doing something to cause them.

On Talking to Your Postpartum Brain

This letter is written to the brain that feels overwhelmed, depleted, lost in the trees, and unfamiliar. The brain that suddenly feels uncertain and detached and scared. Yes, that one. This letter is written to the postpartum brain that has a hold of that mama who is working so hard to see past the fog that is getting in her way of feeling like herself.

Dear Postpartum Brain,

Let me explain what is happening to you so that you feel less afraid, if even momentarily less afraid. There has been an earthquake of sorts. A beautiful baby has been born (and I know that you know this intellectually but simply might not know this with the breath of comforting emotion that you so desire). Along with this beautiful baby is a wave of receding hormones that are affecting your capacity for health and wellness. As that baby left the safety of your belly below, the levels of estrogen and progesterone have dropped significantly in the body that you manage. Those hormones are required for the effective functioning of the parts of you that are required for emotional balance: serotonin, dopamine, and norepinephrine. While some brains find a way to balance back out after this disruption, yours has not.

The imbalance of hormone levels in your body is interfering with your capacity for effective functioning, and so you are left feeling challenged. To put it more simply, the shifting hormone levels are interacting with your chemistry to make you less resilient to stress. While you, Dear Postpartum Brain, once danced beautifully (even while stumbling at times) through periods of stress with relative ease, you are now unable to do so. How frustrating! You suddenly are not able to think clearly and problem solve, as you know. You are suddenly frozen when you were used to flowing freely. You are suddenly more alarmed and anxious about things, and suddenly you are even more in need of feeling in control than you are used to. You, Dear Brain, are being held hostage for the time being.

It is likely that you are getting in the way of your body and your spirit. Those two parts of yourself are now being held hostage by you! I know that you do not mean for this to happen, but your body is tired and depleted and your spirit is crushed. Your body is not being well taken care of by you, and so it is void of energy and nutrients. You are keeping it awake at night. You are quieting its hunger and interfering with its desire to be fed. Your body craves your empathy and your courage and your creativity and your strength so that it can be well. Your body is calling to you. And, because you are not functioning the way you would like to, you are having a hard time answering with ease.

Oh, and your spirit! How much your spirit has been quieted during this siege! Your spirit lacks the energy for company, for social contact, and for familiar love. Your spirit suddenly feels less than, judged, and inadequate. Your spirit is suddenly being taken hold by all of the challenges in its past that it had finally managed to overcome (or so it thought!) because you are unable to think of those challenges with perspective. Your spirit is whispering when it used to sing loud. Your spirit is tentative when it used to be proud. Your spirit is weakened when it used to be strong.

Perhaps you have been here before, Dear Brain, before this beautiful child was born. Perhaps you have once felt this betrayal, and perhaps the birth of this sweet darling baby has sent you back to a place of challenge. My guess is that if you have been here before, you are feeling let down by your own strength to heal. My guess is that if this is all new to you, you are frightened beyond belief because you cannot recognize yourself.

So ... here's the deal. You are not lost forever. Yes, I know you believe that you are, but you most certainly are not. With time and care and effort to heal, you will once again know yourself. You will have the strength and clarity to give your body and your spirit what they need, and you will know—with certainty and with pride—that your beautiful baby is so lucky to have you just as you are. You will know, not just intellectually but also emotionally, that this baby with the soft skin is yours and that you are hers. He will gaze at you with longing and you will gaze back at him with longing in return. No, Postpartum Brain, you are not lost forever.

But, you must get help. I am certain that in most situations you will not just heal on your own with wishful thinking or determination or faking it till you make it. In fact, these strategies are likely to wear you out even more. Most brains under siege like you will need some support that comes from elsewhere—from an empathetic ear, from a medication that will heal your wounds, from some strategic planning around getting you what you need to be well, be it sleep, or food, or love and support. Yes, yes, I know that you want to push through this all by yourself, but why? You are so loved, Dear Postpartum Brain, and you deserve for someone to hold your hand.

I am hopeful that you might feel a bit less lost after reading this letter, or, perhaps, that you might have at least a better sense of why you are feeling so strange. Be kind to the mama who houses you, Dear Postpartum Brain. Be not judgmental but empathetic. Be not unfair but kind. Be not distraught but hopeful. You are still you. And that mama needs you.

Our Nervous Systems in Overdrive

FIGHT, FLIGHT, FREEZE.
REST AND DIGEST.
CONNECT AND PROTECT.
TEND AND BEFRIEND.

Have you heard these terms before? Many of us first heard these jingles in grade school. They have a ring to them and are, dare I say, fun to say. But they are terms that are actually incredibly relevant for many mothers when danger seems to loom in the air for so many. They refer to our **sympathetic** and **parasympathetic** nervous systems, which are the systems that respond to both stress and well-being. When we are afraid, our sympathetic nervous systems are triggered. When we feel safe, our parasympathetic nervous systems are triggered.

Fight and Flight = Sympathetic

Rest and Digest = Parasympathetic

In times of chronic stress, we live in a state of sympathetic overdrive. Many new mothers feel a consistent sense of fear that comes with all of the uncertainty that exists during this time. And in a world that is unpredictable, filled with conflict, and continuing to move through a pandemic, chronic stress is common.

When we are in a state of fear (real or perceived threat and danger), our sympathetic nervous systems kick into gear, and our brains and bodies are thrown into survival mode. Our bodies involuntarily release a force of hormones that trigger our muscles into a state of alertness, affecting heart rates, blood pressure, pupil dilation, body temperature, sweating, and digestion. We feel restless and agitated. We often feel like we can't breathe. Our hearts race. We often can't think straight.

Sound familiar?

However, when we feel safe and secure, our bodies relax their general need to prepare for protection. Our heart rates slow. Our muscles relax. We feel a sense of peace and calm. Our brains are ready to learn and think and absorb information. We are able to rest. And our bodies do their work to heal.

Life is, not surprisingly, threatening right now for many of us as we read the news about the continuing pandemic, war, gun violence, and uncertain rights and respect for vulnerable populations. We feel disconnected and alone and afraid. We are having a major human adventure in unpredictability, inconsistency, and lack of control. Our hearts race. We feel tense. We can't sleep. And we find ourselves in situations where it's suddenly hard to think clearly.

So, we must turn on the parasympathetic nervous system. Like, really turn it on. Intentionally. With effort. Like a warm bath for our nervous systems.

Truthfully, our mental health depends on it.

Many things can trigger this parasympathetic response, and we just need to know what these things are in order to have some influence on our general state of being. But these things aren't hard, and they are actually right at our fingertips. These strategies include the following:

- **Left nostril breathing.** Really. With one hand plug your right nostril and breathe deeply through your left nostril. Long, deep breaths. Try it. This deep breathing technique has been known to quickly settle the nervous system into a state of calm.
- **Meditation.** Yes, I know you know. Always easier said than done though, right? But even if you are someone who believes that "you are not good at meditation," or that "you just can't sit still," the truth is that brain scans show that just three minutes of mindfulness practice can change the nervous system response. If sitting quietly and following your breath is challenging for you, try a guided meditation app like Calm, Insight Timer, or our new favorite, the Mindful Mama app.
- **Connection.** With yourself, others, your environment, or "spirit" (or whatever word works for you with respect to something larger than yourself). And really, even just a moment of connection counts. Try looking someone in the eye. Hugging. Holding a hand. Snuggling with a pet. Walking barefoot outside. Feeling the sun on your face. Planting in a garden. Doing something kind for someone. Feeling your own heartbeat. Talking kindly to yourself. Thanking the Universe (or God, Spirit, Purpose, etc.) for the things you are grateful for. Connect. With something.
- **Do anything, absolutely anything, soothing.** Get a massage. Take a warm bath. Make a cup of tea. Hunker down in child's pose. All of these things will trigger a response in the brain that says "I am safe."

So, a challenge for each of us. Take it or leave it, but, really, if you are finding yourself in a place of chronic tension and stress, you might as well give some attention to that parasympathetic response, just waiting to happen.

Why Is Postpartum Sleep So Important, Anyway?

We all know how important sleep is to our physical health and well-being, but do we really know how much it contributes to our emotional well-being and mental health?

In one of my favorite sleep studies published in the *Archives of Women's Mental Health*, researchers looked at the role that sleep plays in the development of postpartum depression (PPD) in women. They determined that sleep deprivation is an even greater contributing factor in the development of depression and anxiety than the temperament of a baby. In other words, a mom with an "easy" and predictable baby who gets less than four hours of sleep a night is more likely to become and remain depressed than a mom with a colicky baby who gets at least four hours of sleep each night.

Sleep deprivation is used as a torture weapon. The effects that sleep deprivation have on us as humans are extreme. We are less able to think clearly and to make decisions. We become easily overwhelmed. We lose patience and become easily irritated and angry. We stop caring about the things that used to matter to us. We lose interest in the things that usually make us happy, such as exercise, or sex, or social outings, or creativity. We become depressed and sensitive when we used to be carefree, flexible, and happy. In essence, sleep deprivation changes us. It affects who we know ourselves to be. This can be scary.

Yet, as moms, it still seems impossible to change the amount of sleep we get. But look at it this way: As much as we would like to control our babies' temperaments, we can't. And a baby who has colic or who is fussy is often that way despite our best efforts to soothe. As difficult as it is to admit, we often have very little control over this. Our sleep, however, is a different story. We often have more control over the amount of sleep we are getting than we think.

"But how?" you ask. Doesn't a lack of sleep simply come hand in hand with being a new mom? What new mom gets enough sleep, anyway?

All valid and important questions to be asking. In my opinion, while having a baby certainly does make it more difficult to get the amount of sleep we're used to, this does not mean that we need to settle for the inevitable consequences this brings. Each one of us will handle sleep deficiency differently; while some women will adjust accordingly and their bodies will function effectively enough to maintain a baseline of functioning that is adequate, others will not. Women who begin to realize that they are struggling with some of the symptoms of sleep deprivation mentioned above need not simply settle for this as an inevitable part of new parenthood. Will you be getting as much sleep as you did before your baby arrived? Probably not. Is it possible to get enough sleep to aid in preventing PPD and other depressive and anxiety symptoms? Absolutely.

In my work with moms, I encourage them to, whenever possible, make a plan with their partners to share the nighttime duties of having a newborn so as to ensure, for each partner, at least one stint of four hours of uninterrupted sleep a night. For some, this means a short period of sleeping in separate rooms, so that one parent is in a quiet bed for at least a part of the night. For others, this may mean hiring a postpartum doula or night nanny, or inviting a friend or family member to help..

PPD can be debilitating, and it affects not just Mom, but also baby, children, partners, and friends. It is important to think proactively about how you can prevent symptoms of depression and anxiety so you don't struggle more than you need to. Sleep is one of the few things in new motherhood that you do have relative control over, and so thinking through the ways to ensure better sleep is imperative. Athough it's often difficult to recognize, self-care for mom is actually care for baby, too.

Sweet dreams ...

Postpartum Depression and Breastfeeding Challenges: The Connection

Oftentimes, moms come to my practice because of sudden symptoms of postpartum depression or anxiety at the time of weaning from breastfeeding. Some of these moms have chosen to wean; some are weaning because of a milk supply issue, illness, or pain that makes it impossible to continue; and some are weaning because their babies are leading the way. All these moms have been struggling with both breastfeeding and mood challenges that began sometime between birth and their early weaning attempts. All have had questions about whether the breastfeeding and/or the weaning were making them feel worse.

This is not a new trend in my office. As I'm sure it won't surprise you that many women who suffer with a postpartum mood or anxiety disorder like postpartum depression are also struggling through the challenge of breastfeeding. Not all, of course, but many. Some moms who come to my office hold firmly to nursing their babies because it is the one and only thing that they feel is going well. These moms feel strongly that the breastfeeding is getting them through a very difficult emotional time. But I also see a huge number of moms who feel plagued not only by anxiety or depression but also by the fact that breastfeeding is undeniably and unrelentingly difficult. And so it makes them (and me) wonder if the two are connected.

An article in the *Journal of Women's Health* speaks to this very question. In it, the researchers hypothesize that **both mood and lactation might be triggered by the same neuroendocrine mechanisms, or the same hormonal shifts.** We have always known that postpartum depression is a biochemical illness that is triggered by the immense hormonal shifts that occur shortly after birth, and that the ability to breastfeed also depends on effective hormonal activity. But is it possible that the challenges that some moms have with breastfeeding are actually caused by the very same hormonal shifts that leave them feeling sad and anxious?

Following the birth of her baby, a mom's hormones—her estrogen, progesterone, prolactin, thyroid, and cortisol—shift dramatically as her body readjusts from pregnancy to postpartum. These very hormones also have a direct impact on both the brain chemicals that are responsible for emotional wellness and milk production. Sometimes these hormones work together in helping both mood and lactation, and sometimes they work in conflict with the two. Let's break it down as the article did:

PROGESTERONE

Directly following birth, progesterone levels that have been increasing during pregnancy drop dramatically (up to 200 times pre-pregnancy levels) to initiate the start of milk production. When a baby starts to nurse, the suckling stimulates two more hormones, oxytocin and prolactin, which are necessary in let-down and the secretion of milk from a mom's breast. But while this drop in progesterone plays an important part in the production of milk, it also may contribute to the development of a mood disorder because progesterone is required in the maintenance of brain chemistry (in other words, progesterone helps a mom feel emotionally well). So, when it drops? Milk is produced, but some vulnerable moms may also become sad or anxious. (This first-stage hormone shifting is known as the baby blues, but the article mentions that it used to be referred to as "milk fever.") When some moms become anxious or depressed due to the drops in progesterone, the initial challenges with breastfeeding (which are common for most new moms) are more difficult to tolerate because of their symptoms. These moms are simply less resilient to stress.

ESTROGEN

Estrogen levels also drop dramatically, and they remain low throughout lactation. This suggests that low levels of estrogen may be necessary for milk production to occur. But estrogen, like progesterone, is necessary for brain chemical balance (it has a direct impact on serotonin, the "feel good hormone"), and so the same conflict might occur: Low estrogen, which is necessary for breastfeeding, may also lead some women to develop symptoms of postpartum depression and/or anxiety. Again, these moms may have a harder time working through early feeding challenges because of their symptoms.

OXYTOCIN

Oxytocin is that lovely hormone that leads to feelings of pleasure, comfort, and maternal security. In fact, it has been said that oxytocin is responsible for the onset of early maternal behaviors that lead mothers (both human and animals) to instinctively protect their little ones. Oxytocin production also stimulates let-down in the breastfeeding mama. Some studies have suggested that moms who are depressed or anxious during pregnancy have lower levels of oxytocin. And, yup, you got it, if these moms have less oxytocin, they are also likely to have challenges with let-down and may also not feel that initial sense of connection to their babes. So these same moms who are depressed or anxious while pregnant are likely to have additional struggles when attempting to breastfeed after their babes are born.

PROLACTIN

Prolactin levels increase in a mom's body during pregnancy and the early postpartum period. Over time, baseline prolactin levels drop, but each time a baby suckles, prolactin levels are increased briefly for milk production to be stimulated. Prolactin is also thought to play a role in the emotional wellness of a new mom as both animal and human studies have found that high prolactin triggers a maternal response in the caretaking of a baby (feeding, keeping safe, attentiveness). On the other spectrum, it has been found in some studies that women who have low levels of prolactin during pregnancy are prone to higher levels of anxiety. It also seems that high levels of stress can interfere with the mechanisms for prolactin release in women. So ... low prolactin may lead to both anxiety and low milk supply, which may lead to high stress, which may lead to low prolactin and low milk supply, which may lead to high stress and anxiety, which may lead to ...

THYROID

As many as five percent of women will develop a thyroid imbalance postpartum. And some studies have found a link between low thyroid levels and poor milk supply. Low thyroid levels (also known as hypothyroid) have also been shown to induce depressive symptoms in women. If a mama has an imbalance in her thyroid levels after birth, she may find that both her milk production and her mood are affected.

CORTISOL

During pregnancy, a stress hormone known as cortisol increases. After childbirth, these cortisol levels typically drop, and do so even more dramatically in healthy breastfeeding moms (this contributes to the feeling of calm and well-being while nursing that some breastfeeding moms describe). Successful milk production and let-down involve an adequate circulation of cortisol, and it seems that when cortisol levels are not balanced out appropriately, both milk production and mood can be affected: Higher cortisol levels are linked to higher levels of anxiety and stress. Moms who are anxious postpartum probably have higher levels of cortisol while breastfeeding, which may interfere with milk production and make it so that she does not experience the good feelings that are so often assumed to relate to nursing.

So, what does all this mean for you? What it means is that, if you are having difficulties postpartum—whether with depression or anxiety symptoms or with breastfeeding—it is not your fault. None of it. You are not anxious or depressed because you are not trying hard enough or because you are not doing something right. You are also not having a hard time with breastfeeding because you are failing at something. Our bodies go through one heck of a roller-coaster ride after our babies are born, and some women's bodies (many, actually) are just less tolerant of this amusement park of sorts. Some of us simply don't like roller coasters.

Mindfulness Meditation Practice and the Brain: Why It Matters in Motherhood

Don't worry, I'm not going to tell you that you need to create an altar, light a candle every morning, sit cross-legged for an hour, or become a Zen master.

Though of course if those things call out to you, be my guest—they might serve your mental health and wellness in some way.

What I do want you to know is that the science reminds us, over and over, that a regular mindfulness practice changes our brains and creates opportunity for calm, connection, and distress tolerance. If you are reading this book, you know that having more of those things would be helpful. You are likely out of practice.

For most of us, and without regular practice, our thoughts run the show. Our thinking moves from what has happened in the past to what might happen in the future. We have an experience of regret or uncertainty, and our bodies feel tight or unsettled or numb. In these frequent instances, if someone asks us a question, we might not hear them accurately. We are less likely to pay attention to the small details. We act in ways that we later regret. Our non-present mind takes away from what matters most: what is happening now.

Our reaction to past regret and future uncertainty is, quite frankly, a villain in this story. It's the reaction that brings with it *discomfort* and likes to take over. When this happens, we get lost in its energy.

When that villain enters the scene, it's so hard to be still! So many of us have developed the habit of doing. Doing the dishes. Doing the parenting. Doing the organizing. Doing the planning. Doing the talking. Doing the thinking. Doing the fixing. *Doing it all.* Yes, of course there is much to do—you are a mom after all—but many of us keep moving and doing because when we actually slow down, we *feel*. As you will keep hearing over and over in this book, many of us are not taught how to really feel and, instead, are taught that any moment of emotional discomfort means that something is wrong.

You will keep hearing here that discomfort is not a problem.

So, what is mindfulness practice? Why does it matter? Mindfulness meditation practice includes the following:

1. *Stillness and quiet*
2. *Reflection*
3. *Engaging in a repetitive and focused exercise such as concentration on one's breathing or repetition of a mantra, for the purpose of reaching a heightened level of present-moment awareness.*

This practice teaches us to stay with what *is*, right here in the *moment*. We learn not to distract or run away or think ourselves out of what is happening *now*. Right now, right in this very moment, you are okay. You always have been, and you always will be. Even in times of stress or pain or emotional challenge or uncertainty. In the moment, you are okay. But we must be *mindful* to be in the moment.

You getting the drift?

Important and clinically sound research has proved over and over that mindfulness meditation practice is especially beneficial for people (that means you, moms) who struggle with depression, anxiety, and chronic pain. What these studies are showing is that changes in brain activity in people who have learned to meditate hold steady even when they're not meditating. What does that mean for you? It means that after a short practice (let's say just 5 to 10 minutes) in mindfulness-based meditation, you are likely to continue to remain steady, in the moment, tolerant to stress and discomfort, and less engaged with your thoughts for the rest of the day.

For the rest of the day!

You see, in mindfulness practice, we learn to accept the rambling thoughts rather than engage with them. We learn to accept the physiological impacts of emotional distress rather than needing to get rid of them. We learn to ground ourselves in the here and now rather than getting pulled away from the moment by those reactions to regret and uncertainty.

We learn to stay *here*.

Because, usually, the *here*—even the more challenging emotions and feelings—just comes with the territory of being a human. Of being a mom. Find me a mother who doesn't have a zillion moments of discomfort and uncertainty, and I'll give you a million dollars.

For the neuroscience buffs like me who are reading, here are some important things to know from the research:

- Long-term meditators (those folks who have a regular and ongoing practice in meditation) have longer-lasting gray matter in their brains as they age. These well-preserved brains are sharper.
- Mindfulness meditation helps with that annoying monkey-brain that many of us have by limiting activity in the default mode network (DMN), which triggers mind-wandering and thoughts about ourselves and the external world around us. As I know you know, these types of thoughts will lead us toward worrying about the past and future, which, inevitably, impacts our sense of happiness and well-being.
- Meditation can even change the structure of the brain! Studies that followed courses in mindfulness-based stress reduction (MBSR) found that two important parts of participants' brains actually increased in thickness. The hippocampus (which regulates learning and memory) and areas of the brain

that play roles in emotion regulation actually both get *bigger!* And these same studies showed that for regular practitioners, the amygdala (where fear, anxiety, and stress is born) actually *decreased* in size. The amygdala got *smaller*!

- Meditation supports the parts of the brain responsible for concentration and attention.
- Mindfulness-based meditation practices have long-lasting impacts on stress reduction. For example, research showed us that after just one 8-week class in mindfulness-based stress reduction, participants reported a reduction in stress for *years* afterward.

Are you convinced yet?

I know it can feel daunting to start a practice in mindfulness and meditation, but I'm pretty sure it's worth a try. Here are some important places to start:

1. Find a quiet place with as few distractions as possible. (A bathroom? Closet? Extra room where the door closes? Corner of your bedroom?)
2. Find a comfortable posture. (Make it comfortable! Sit, lie down, put your feet up the wall. Whatever works.)
3. Find a focus for your attention (such as a specific word that you say over and over, the sensation of your breath, or a candle).
4. Do not judge yourself for anything that happens, and be open to whatever happens. If you get caught up in your thoughts, notice this and let go and come back to the focus of your attention. If you are uncomfortable, shift your body and then come back to your attention. If a fly is buzzing around your head or you hear children crying in the other room—assuming they are supervised—let those agitations be there, and then come back to the focus of your attention.

Does it sound hard? You're in luck—it's supposed to be hard. Please don't buy into those myths that meditation practice should feel good or that good meditators have quiet and calm minds. Nope, not true. It's the process of practice with those things that matters, not whether or not those things are occurring.

I've had a regular meditation practice for years, and I still feel agitated and distracted every time I sit down.

But it works. I feel better.

And it makes me a better mom.

III. PSYCHOLOGICAL HEALTH
Your Beliefs, Thoughts & Feelings

The Dilemma about Control

Let me start with the punchline:

The only two things that humans actually have control over are their own thoughts and their own behaviors.

That's it. We influence other things for sure. But we absolutely do not have control over anything else. Not the weather. Not the political landscape. Not the ebbs and flows of viruses and bacteria. We don't have control over when our children will sleep. We can't control when or what our children eat. We don't have control over our partners', family members', friends', or neighbors' moods, preferences, or opinions. We can't control what, exactly, will happen when we give birth or how, exactly, we will feel when we look at our babies for the first time. We can't control the temperament of our children or the annoying shit that our partners do. We can't even, believe it or not, control our feelings.

What we do have control over is simply (*don't get that word confused with "easily," but more on that later*) how we think about or respond to these things. That's it. Think about all that time we are wasting trying to control and manipulate the people and environments around us. So much effort, energy, and commitment spent trying to control things that are *outside* of our control. It's exhausting, isn't it? We feel so dang out of control all the time. Still. We push and we pull, and we hope, and we expect, and we tire ourselves in the process. We are usually, if not always, disappointed in the end.

But our agency—the place where we really do have control—lies within ourselves, rather than outside of us. When we slow way down and pause and take a moment to make a choice that has to do with what we are thinking or how we are behaving, we have a sudden sense of being grounded and stable. Just for a moment.

Our own thoughts and our own behaviors.

I'm telling you; it feels good.

WE CHOOSE TO SAY SOMETHING KIND TO OURSELVES RATHER THAN TRY TO CONTROL WHAT OTHERS ARE SAYING TO US.

WE CHOOSE TO BREATHE DEEPLY RATHER THAN TRY TO GET OTHER PEOPLE TO CALM DOWN.

WE CHOOSE TO SPEAK ABOUT HOW WE FEEL RATHER THAN TELLING SOMEONE HOW THEY SHOULD FEEL.

WE CHOOSE TO OFFER THE MILK OR THE FOOD OR THE WATER RATHER THAN YELLING AT OUR CHILDREN FOR NOT DRINKING OR EATING WHEN WE WANT THEM TO.

WE CHOOSE TO FOCUS ON HOW WE CREATE BEDTIME ROUTINES, HOW WE SETTLE OUR OWN NERVOUS SYSTEMS BEFORE WE SLEEP TRAIN, AND HOW TO SET BOUNDARIES AROUND WHAT WE ARE AND ARE NOT WILLING TO DO WHEN IT COMES TO NIGHTTIME RITUALS. WE FOCUS ON THESE THINGS RATHER THAN TRYING TO CONTROL WHEN OUR CHILDREN ACTUALLY (FINALLY) CLOSE THEIR EYES. (AND BOY OH BOY, WE ALL KNOW THAT NEVER WORKS.)

WE CHOOSE HOW TO SETTLE OURSELVES WHEN WE ARE SCARED, ANGRY, SAD, OR DISAPPOINTED RATHER THAN TRYING OH SO DESPERATELY (AND INEFFECTIVELY) TO CONTROL THE THINGS THAT ARE CAUSING OUR FEAR, ANGER, OR SADNESS.

Are you getting the point? It is in *these* moments that we have control. When we have control, we settle. Just like that!

This is a simple concept. **Instead of trying to control all the things that are outside of us, we can shift and put all that effort back into controlling what we can: ourselves.** But this concept is far from easy. As a generalization, humans do not like to *not* be in control, and so letting go of those things that we so desperately want to believe are ours to manipulate is really hard. It's terrifying. And when we are scared, we are wired to protect. We grip and hold on tightly. We try even harder to gain control over what isn't ours. But the reality is that even though not being in control of something feels like a threat, it likely is not. Not being in control of something is uncomfortable for sure. It is incredibly inconvenient. But the fact of *not* having control over many things in life isn't, typically, dangerous.

So, just to nail it down, let's play a game for a moment. Grab a pen and paper or talk out loud. Answer this question: *What do I absolutely not have any control over?*

Hint: My children's interests and opinions, my children's biological clocks, my husband's choices around his work schedule, former President Trump's behavior, my neighbor's loudly barking dog, the spotty internet in Boulder, my family of origin's opinions about the choices that I make, my colleague's disappointment about something that I said no to, the natural aging that occurs in my body as I near 50, my teenager's moodiness, the ups and downs of the COVID pandemic.

Okay. How do you feel? What do you notice in your body? Are you tense? Agitated? Short of breath?

And now, ask yourself this question: *What do I have control over?*

Hint: How deep of a breath I take. Whether or not I pause before speaking. The words I use to talk to my partner about how I feel when he works late. The choices I make to act in support of women's rights and equality and peace in the world. Whether or not to wear earplugs at night so that the barking dog doesn't keep me up. Ways to have humor about the (incredibly annoying) telehealth blunders during a pandemic. The ways in which I remind myself that my job is to be loyal to myself and that I can't make everyone happy. Drinking enough water to take care of my body and skin and brain. Finding other mothers who have had similar experiences to talk to about the challenges of raising teenage daughters. Wearing a mask, washing my hands, and giving myself permission to feel it all.

Now? When you realize where your control lies, and when you realize that it is right at your fingertips, do you feel a shift? Does something move? Can you breathe a bit deeper?

It's worth a try, dear readers. Don't just take my word for it; ask yourself if this applies to you. *Do you actually have any realistic control over the things outside of you that you are working so hard to change? Are you frustrated and exhausted from trying? Do you find that you continue to feel* out *of control even when you put limitless effort and energy into trying to control those things, time and time again?*

If this is true of you, too, see what happens when you shift your energy, just a little bit, to what you actually do have control over. Those little thoughts and behaviors are cumulative. I can almost guarantee you that you will begin to feel more in control over time.

Oh, and by the way, I need to practice all this stuff too. We all do.

When We Are Scared, We Get Scary

Several basic human emotions exist for all of us. Frequently, these are thought to be the following: happiness, sadness, disgust, fear, and anger.

And *anger*, oh *anger*. Many of us, especially if we are women, have been taught that anger is bad. Not okay. Something to be avoided. Something to resist or push down or hide from.

But what if I told you that anger was hardwired to protect you? What if I told you that anger is the emotion that shows up when you feel fear? What if I told you that the truth is that *when all humans are scared, they get scary*, and anger is the exhibition of this fear? That while anger can seem gruff and mean and big, it comes from a very, very tender human place. That all anger stems from fear. **Scary people are, well, scared.**

We've all seen it in real time: *Your kiddo runs toward the street, and you scream at him to stop. Someone treats your kiddo poorly, and you become mama bear, whipping out your sharp tongue and your fierce protection. You are giving birth and you feel anger toward the people around you who don't seem to be helping. Your partner does something that leaves you feeling unseen and alone and you lash out. Your teenager is pushing you away and you get angry in return.*

Fear.

When we are scared, we get scary.

Sometimes this is not as obvious, like when a person in power gets mean and violent. But it is there at its core even then.

But why is this important, you ask? It's important because when we communicate from a place of anger, we often unintentionally push people farther away. What we all want is closeness and connection; we are hardwired for this. So, when we feel any sort of injustice or abandonment or rejection coming from the people around us (our children, our partner, our family, our friends, our community, society), we armor ourselves up to fight. To protect ourselves. While this is the case some of the time for sure, very often we are not actually in danger. We are afraid, but we don't need to fight.

What we need is to connect.

So, the takeaway is this: **Acknowledge and communicate your fear when you can.**

"Mommy is worried that you might get hurt."

"I am feeling scared that you might leave."

"I feel fear when I don't know if you are paying attention/listening to me."

"It feels scary to feel invisible."

"I am feeling worried that you don't trust that I am here for you."

Let me be clear. I do believe that anger serves a purpose, and that like all other emotions, anger holds immense wisdom: *Something is happening here that is not okay.* But what if you learned to communicate from the tenderness of fear rather than the sharpness of anger?

Next time you are feeling angry, ask yourself this:

What am I afraid of?

See if you can pause and connect from that place.

How Wishing Postpartum Depression Away Can Hinder Your Recovery

We do lots of strategy building in my psychotherapy practice. This is an important part of the work for women as they move toward wellness in the postpartum period. At the same time, in the work that I do, attention is paid to a very careful balance between the "being" and the "doing" pieces involved in recovery from a postpartum mood or anxiety disorder like postpartum depression. Often, women want nothing more than to get themselves the heck out of where they are—both emotionally and logistically.

"I cannot feel like this for one more second," so many of these moms say. "I want out," they acknowledge. "I want to just get on a bus and disappear," they determine. "I should have never decided to have children," they mourn. "I do not want to have to be in this therapy office," they declare.

Oh, how much I wish I could push that big, red, shiny button for these mamas and make all the pain and suffering disappear. That would be so wonderfully simple and such a relief. Being in that place of great despair is so heart-wrenching and conflicting for the women who find themselves there.

Acknowledging this place of great hurt is difficult. But it is also an important part of the recovery process. Wishing it all away is a natural reaction but also is, quite frankly, self-defeating. Most of us will find that the more we try to feel differently, the less likely we are to move in that direction. Instead, and against all that seems rational now, meeting yourself right where you are during postpartum depression or anxiety is the place from which all recovery stems.

Instead of judging ourselves for our shortcomings, we try to validate. Instead of telling ourselves it is wrong to feel a certain way, we empathize. Instead of getting out the punching bag, we muster up a hug. For ourselves.

With all the amazing and empowering gifts that motherhood offers, being a mom is also bloody hard work—especially if you are struggling with a perinatal mood or anxiety disorder like postpartum depression. It is backbreaking. It is heartbreaking. It is confusing. It is exhausting. It is overwhelming. It is draining. It sometimes feels suffocating. It requires us to face our shortcomings. It asks us to be willing to make mistakes. It beckons us to revisit old hurts. It pushes us to look at who we are and where we have been. All of this can catch moms off guard when the most "expected" thing is maternal bliss and happiness. Yes, this happens too, but often not for quite some time for many women.

There is a difference here, I must add, between meeting yourself where you are with acceptance, compassion, and understanding and "settling in" to this uncomfortable place as a way of giving in to the power of these challenges. I am not asking you to give up or to hand yourself over or to decide that this is how you will feel forever. I am asking you to simply open yourself up to what is happening for you as a way of looking it straight in the eye as if to say, *"Okay. Here I am. I see you despair/anxiety/overwhelm/sadness. I am looking at you for what you are, and I am now going to hug myself, hold my own hand, and do my best to close the door on your company."*

Understanding Vulnerability in Motherhood

What comes to mind when you hear the word "vulnerability"? What are the images, words, and reactions that invite themselves along with that word? My guess is that it is something like this: *weakness, fear, shame, powerlessness, and insecurity.* I imagine that, for most of you, the word "vulnerability" sends with it a warning sign and a very deafening message of "Be Tough!" I imagine that all of you reading this know what it feels like to be vulnerable and that most of you are working very, very hard to run in the opposite direction. To prove to others that you are anything but.

I am reminded of professor and author Brené Brown's phenomenal research on vulnerability. Her message is that to feel strong, empowered, and connected, we must face vulnerability head-on. Not run from it or resist it. Her decade of research tells us that the people who run from vulnerability are the ones who continue to feel shame, a lack of worthiness, and fear, and that the people who embrace vulnerability are the ones who feel worthy, connected, and strong. It is somewhat counterintuitive, isn't it? This conclusion may confuse many of us who have been taught, from an early age, that admitting to vulnerability is failure. But this conclusion may, when all is said and done, provide postpartum moms some freedom.

For most women who walk into my office, *vulnerability* is assumed to be a dirty word. For the first-time therapy client, the brand-new mom, or the woman who exists in a place of shame and unworthiness, vulnerability is to be avoided at all costs. The idea of it is terrifying. For many people, it equates with failure. It suggests lack of competence. This resistance takes charge of the mom who is suffering in silence and is terrified to ask for help because she assumes this means she is weak. This gets expressed in my office as, "I feel so much shame for having to be here. I feel like I should be able to do this without any help."

But yet that mom is there, in my office. That mom *is* vulnerable. Not because she is weak, but because she is a mom. And she is human.

Let's, just for a moment, name all of the times in early motherhood that we are vulnerable:

When we try to get pregnant; when we learn that we are pregnant; during the first trimester; when we experience miscarriage; when we become pregnant again; when our bodies change before our eyes; when we give birth; when we adopt a child; when we attempt to breastfeed our babies; when we choose to bottle-feed our babies; when we wean; when we bring our babies home from the hospital, when our midwives leave, or when we bring our adopted babies home for the first time; when our babies cry; when we don't have the answers; when we make mistakes; when we experience our partners' struggle; when we are tired; when we are hungry; when we forget to change a diaper and our babies get a rash; when we lose our temper; when our feelings are hurt; when we realize we have hurt someone else's feelings; when we are trying to cook dinner, tend to a newborn, and manage our toddler's tantrums or endless chatter all at once; when we burn the toast; when we don't recognize our bodies; when we have sex with our partners; when we don't want to have sex with our partners; when we are cold; when we are hot; when we are lonely; when we are sad; when our hormones are shifting; when we are surprised by something; when we are disappointed by something; when our expectations aren't met.... Get it?

WE FEEL VULNERABLE ALL THE TIME.

What many of us do is this: panic. We assume that if we are vulnerable, something must be wrong with us. We pretend to feel invincible when we aren't. We say that we are fine when we're not. We refuse help when we need it. We attempt to be who we aren't in that moment: We pretend to be moms who are superhuman and impenetrable.

What would it mean if being "strong" meant knowing our limits and asking for help when we need it? What if being worthy meant understanding our own individual challenges and working with them rather than against them? What if being competent meant being super-duper authentic with where we are emotionally, physically, and spiritually in each and every moment? What if being okay meant being willing to not be okay? What if the ability to acknowledge vulnerability was a strength and not a weakness?

Well, what Brené Brown's research says is this: We would be happier. It says that we would feel more connected to others. It says that we would report more feelings of worthiness and less shame. It says that we would feel more competent, more capable, and more in control. It says that by simply "leaning in" to discomfort, we will be freed of the burden of it. Imagine that!

Postpartum mood and anxiety disorders like PPD have many layers to them. Moms who struggle with depression and anxiety often are dealing with a double whammy of vulnerability: They are vulnerable both because they are moms and because the symptoms associated with depression and anxiety are making it hard for them to think with clarity and confidence. These moms may want nothing more than to wish their vulnerabilities away because they feel awful. But the more they try to not be vulnerable, the more they feel that they are. They feel shame, and guilt, and worthlessness. And they resist these feelings of vulnerability. And around, and around, and around.

If Brené Brown's 10+ years of research is accurate, we know with a fair amount of certainty that this resistance to vulnerability and this assumption that being vulnerable is a character flaw only causes more distress and creates a deeper sense of isolation and lack of needed connection. If we understand this, then we all may want to try something new: We may want to take a deep breath, find our inner courage and strength, and let someone in on our little secret. Reach out for help. Give ourselves permission to be vulnerable simply because we are. My guess is that by doing this, we get what we need to feel better.

The Ands and Buts of Postpartum Depression

Let's give something a try. I invite you to say each of the statements below.

Out loud.

1. I love my new baby, *but* I just don't enjoy the responsibility of caring for a newborn.
2. I love my new baby, *and* I just don't enjoy the responsibility of caring for a newborn.

Do you feel a difference within yourself when you say this same idea two different ways? Which statement is accompanied by feelings of failure, guilt, and shame? Which is accompanied by some acceptance, empathy, and understanding?

It helps to know the difference between Either/Or and Both/And.

"*Either* I love my baby, *or* I don't like the logistics of being a new mom" versus "I *both* love my new baby *and* don't enjoy the logistics of being a new mom." You see, most women who are struggling with postpartum depression or a related illness go into that "either/or" place that is inevitably associated with feelings of guilt, self-doubt, shame, and failure. To these moms, either you love your baby and every minute of childcare and mothering, *or* you don't like the early weeks and months as much as you thought you would and therefore this must mean that you don't love your baby as much as you should, and you are a terrible mother.

I would bet that the above statement is a belief and *not* a truth.

Language and the ways we talk to ourselves have immense power over the way we feel. When we use the word "but," it seems to cancel out everything before it, whereas the word "and" allows for some acceptance and a bigger picture of the truth. The word "and" allows for the important credit that you deserve. It allows for your strengths and not just your challenges. It invites understanding and perspective. It brings hope.

The word "but"? It cancels out everything before it. It shuts down the conversation. It closes hope, and it assumes that things won't change. It creates a big wall around compromise and acceptance. It really doesn't serve us one bit.

So I would bet that these are the statements that make the most sense:

I have always wanted to be a mama, ***and*** *this is not what I expected.*

My baby has these moments of sweetness, ***and*** *it is really difficult to tolerate it when she cries.*

I want what's best for my baby, ***and*** *I don't think that I want to continue attempting to breastfeed him.*

I have always thought of myself as a strong and competent woman, ***and*** *I can't do this alone.*

I labored for several hours naturally, ***and*** *I got an epidural.*

I know that I need to take care of myself, ***and*** *the logistics around this seem really complicated.*

I want to ask for help, ***and*** *I am worried about what others might think if they know I am struggling.*

So, I leave you with a challenge today, an invitation to be mindful of the way you talk to yourself and others about your experiences. Every time you catch yourself moving toward a "yeah, but...," take a deep breath. Reevaluate. Trade that impulse for a "yes, and..." It takes practice, and it also makes a world of difference.

Getting Rid of the Guilt

We have all felt it at one time or another: guilt. It is a word that you will find everywhere in almost anything that is written to, for, or about mothers.

"Mommy guilt" they call it.

"It is just part of the game," I have heard people say. Bloggers, journalists, and TV writers say all the time that motherhood simply comes with guilt. Moms feel guilty that they can't give enough, do enough, and be enough to everyone who needs them all the time.

Okay, so if moms who are functioning to capacity feel guilt, what about the mom who has struggled with a postpartum mood disorder like postpartum depression?

Sure, these moms feel guilty about not having the energy to play as they imagined. They feel guilty for being irritable toward their spouse, partner, baby, or children. They feel guilty that they haven't done the laundry in weeks and the house is a mess. They feel guilty that they have not returned phone calls and emails or sent thank-you notes. They feel guilty that they are serving frozen pizza and mac-n-cheese instead of the home-cooked meals they imagined. They feel guilty for getting an epidural, or not breastfeeding, or not enjoying teeny tiny diapers at three in the morning. They feel guilty for wanting to go back to work. Or for wanting to stay at home. They feel guilty for not wanting to have sex. For wanting to take breaks. For taking breaks. And for wanting and needing childcare support.

But on top of all of these "shortcomings," moms with postpartum depression feel guilty that they aren't meeting societal norms about motherhood. In their deepest and darkest places, they feel guilty about being so miserable at a time when moms are told they "should" feel unmatched joy, bonding, and enlightenment in motherhood.

For moms with PPD, guilt is a symptom that is often the last to be remedied. That's *a lot* of guilt.

Guilt can quickly turn to shame, and shame is both a curious and devastatingly destructive emotion. It lingers. It takes up space. So often it creeps in with such force that it begins to define us. We feel inadequate, flawed, unworthy, and damaged. Our guilt-turned-to-shame crushes us. With that, it creates an invisible but **very** visceral wall between us and the people we love.

In my practice, I talk extensively with my clients about emotions, their role, and their importance in our lives. As difficult as feeling emotion can be, it does serve a purpose. So if this is true, what on Earth is the purpose of a not-so-friendly emotion like guilt?

On a good day, guilt lets us know that we have done something wrong, and propels us to make amends, fix our mistakes, and do better next time. Guilt helps us gain a better sense of who we want to be and invites us to reexamine our choices and our behavior so that we don't make the same mistake twice. When it is serving its purpose, guilt can lead us to repair the mistakes that we make, which, according to influential pediatrician and psychoanalyst Donald Winnicott, actually makes us better mothers.

But on a bad day, when guilt verges on shame, it can be unhealthy and inappropriate. On these days, we are frozen by our guilt, and we either don't move to repair or we aren't satisfied when we do. On these days, guilt lingers and steals our attention away from the things that we want to be doing and the people (namely our babies) whom we want so desperately to love. It is in these instances that we believe we are punishing ourselves (because, well, so many of us believe that we should). But, instead, we are continuing to punish those around us by making ourselves unavailable to the moment.

So, what can we do about this? What can we do if that lingering guilt just won't get off our backs? What can we do if our postpartum depression has exited the center stage, but it leaves its sidekick guilt in the picture?

First, I invite you to ask yourself this question: What is *within my control that I can do to alleviate this feeling of guilt?* If you come up with something, do it: apologize to your spouse, your toddler, or your newborn. Decide whether or not it is important for you to disclose information about your illness to family, friends, coworkers, and neighbors so that they understand why you have been distant, unavailable, less than productive, or less than friendly. Write a group email and thank your support team and community for being there. And then, **forgive yourself**.

Yes, I know, easier said than done.

For this challenge, I ask you this: Is what you are feeling actually guilt? Is it directed at you? Are you feeling this way because you have committed a wrong? Are you, indeed, guilty as charged?

Or is what you are feeling more likely regret?

I ask because the word makes a difference. The Merriam-Webster dictionary defines guilt as "*the fact of having committed a breach of conduct especially violating law and involving a penalty.*" It defines regret as "*to mourn the loss of*" and "*to be very sorry for.*" My guess is that if you really explore this question, you will find that what you are feeling is not guilt, but rather regret.

You regret that you were not able to breastfeed; you mourn the loss of this experience. You regret that you did not enjoy the early weeks or months of parenting; you mourn the loss of expectation. You regret that you were irritable with the people you love; you feel sorry about this.

When you exchange the word "guilt" for "regret," its definition takes the need for punishment away. Instead of insisting that you must be locked up and condemned for something, you simply allow yourself to be sad about an event, time, or situation that was missed. Believe it or not, sadness is often a much more manageable emotion to tolerate.

Moms, you are certainly allowed to regret having struggled during pregnancy or postpartum. Instead of being harmful, allowing yourself to be sad about this might also help you to move on.

When Negative Beliefs Become Truths: On Self-Doubt

There's quite an amazing thing that happens in my psychotherapy practice week after week with moms who have postpartum depression: Themes emerge. Truly.

Sometimes almost every mother I see is struggling with communication with her partner. Another week, the dance for nearly everyone I see is to the tune of the need for self-care and the seeming impossibility of this endeavor. One week I may have a handful of mamas wondering "where they went" once they became mothers and who are struggling with the overwhelming task of deciding who they would like to be. The next week, mom after mom is treading through the past to better understand her own experience in childhood so that she might have the courage to pave new roadways for her own children.

Some weeks each mom is in tears. Other weeks laughter abounds. Sometimes it seems that the common topic is medication and the often-complicated conversation about whether this choice feels appropriate. Other times the sessions abound with referrals to acupuncturists, psychiatrists, support groups, and nutritionists.

I mention this tendency for themes as a reminder that so often what you think you alone are struggling with while going through postpartum depression or anxiety is happening to the many women you pass on the street on your way here or there. These challenges are real. For many, many, many women.

One common theme? Beliefs. Not beliefs in the spiritual or religious sense, but the beliefs that become truths for so many women who are struggling during pregnancy or postpartum. One mom in my office *believes* that having a baby means that life is destroyed. One mom *believes* that she is not a good mom because she was unable to breastfeed. One mom *believes* that she should be happy because she has a healthy baby and a family who loves her. One mom *believes* that she should not take time for herself because "good mothers" want to be with their children all the time. One mom *believes* that she must be crazy and awful because she is having terrifying intrusive thoughts that she knows are wrong but she cannot turn off. One mom *believes* that she will be an unfit mother because she dislikes being pregnant and is not the glowing model of happiness as her belly grows.

I could go on. These themes are not only about beliefs but also about intense struggle for the women I see: of tears, frustration, and seemingly limitless self-doubt.

This is a place where it's important to look at thought patterns and the way they intrude in our ability to feel hopeful about ourselves and our situations. You see, when the conversation begins to unfold, it becomes a bit clearer that while each mom claims her belief to be a truth, the reality is not so.

Millions of spectacular mothers are unable to breastfeed or choose not to breastfeed. Rooms exist that are full of women whose postpartum period is challenged by depression and/or anxiety and who have healthy children and loving families.

I think I can safely say that not one mother out there, whether or not she is struggling with a perinatal mood or anxiety disorder like postpartum depression, wants to be with her children all the time, and moms who take time to fulfill their own needs away from the demands of parenthood will undoubtedly have so much more to give their children for it.

Quite truthfully, the idea that every woman who is pregnant is a glowing model of happiness and optimism is a myth that I wish I could crush on the spot.

Beliefs are like well-tread pathways. They come from somewhere deep inside and long ago, and they can literally color the way that we all look at the world and at ourselves. They come from experiences, from messages our parents gave us, from society, and from the often unrealistically high standards we set for ourselves. Over time, these beliefs become so true to us that the line between belief and truth becomes blurred and tangled. When we aren't paying attention, we will often take these individual and very personal beliefs as facts. While this is a universal phenomenon, it is also a dangerous one as when we make this mistake, we unconsciously close ourselves off from all other perspectives. Our brains' confirmation bias will, literally, stop paying attention to any evidence that goes against what we believe to be true. Suddenly we have created a world for ourselves that we don't want at all.

The mom who thinks that having a baby means that her life is destroyed most likely has a valid reason for believing this. But it is helpful to ask where this belief came from; where did she learn this, and is it possible that this isn't a truth at all and that with support and hard work she can create a new belief for herself?

Yes, if only a magic button existed and we could all push it to make things change instantly, to suddenly see things differently and create new truths for ourselves just like that. That button would be well-worn, let me tell you.

No, none of this is as easy as that, I know. But beliefs can change. They do, even without big, red, shiny buttons. The journey through postpartum depression recovery, and that of related illnesses, takes us through many different places, and it is important to remember that you really do get to choose what you want to believe to be true. For yourself and for your little ones.

What were/are the beliefs that you had/have that influenced the way you felt about yourself and mothering?

How Your Own Mother and Childhood Trauma Can Impact Your Maternal Mental Health

You have just given birth to a baby whom you have been waiting anxiously to meet. Even if you are someone whose pregnancy was not ideal, it is likely that you have been holding on to the hope that when you meet this baby on the outside, many of the discomforts or insecurities you've been feeling will dissipate. You know the drill: "When I pass through the first trimester ... when I hit the 37-week mark ... when this baby is born ... things will get better."

You finally do get to meet this little one face-to-face and then, out of nowhere, comes a sudden panic: *"What if I can't do this? What if I am just like my mother? I don't have a road map for this that I feel comfortable with!"* Or, for others: *"What if I can't be enough like my own mom?"* For some mamas, this may look different. For some, meeting baby for the first time brings great joy and excitement, and it is later, when the adrenaline wears off, that the stuff from childhood creeps in.

This can happen to anyone, regardless of whether you think of your childhood as conflicted. New moms who have wonderfully secure relationships with their own parents can suddenly feel the ripple of ambivalence creep in when their own babies are born.

Early childhood trauma experiences are often the most unexpected risk factor for developing a postpartum mood or anxiety disorder like postpartum depression. With the increasing information on perinatal mood and anxiety disorders (PMADs), many women now anticipate the bumps that come with hormone changes, identity shifting, and breastfeeding challenges. But few new moms anticipate the emotional turbulence that can accompany old memories when they resurface.

The hardest part about this is that you may not always be aware of where some of your emotion is coming from ... and so what is an older feeling or memory that is being triggered can appear as an emotion or a challenge in the present.

Let me explain this with an example:

A mom comes into my office because she is feeling anxious, overwhelmed, and helpless when caring for her newborn baby. When this baby cries, she is overcome by feelings of worthlessness. She gets angry with her daughter for not nursing better. For not sleeping more. For not "loving her." And then, this mom is filled with guilt for these feelings. "I must be a terrible mother for thinking these things!" she says. "I just can't do this!"

Through further assessment, it becomes clear that this mama never really felt heard or validated for how she was feeling when she, herself, was a kiddo. If she came home feeling sad because another kid bullied her at school, she was told to "stop crying and be a big girl." When she fell and scraped a knee, she was told to "shake it off." When she crawled into her parents' room late at night, scared of the dark, she was expected to "stop being such a scaredy-cat." In short, this woman was always told that she shouldn't feel the way she was feeling, and that showing emotion was simply not okay.

Now she has become a mom herself. And guess what? She is unsure of how to respond when her own baby cries. Truthfully, why should she be sure? It is amazing to me how we all expect ourselves to know exactly what to do in moments of stress even if we haven't been taught how to do this. If a mom wasn't validated and empathized with by someone in her life when she was a child, how can we expect her to know how to do this with her baby? Just as importantly, how can we expect her to empathize with and validate herself in these moments of difficulty?

Of course, the examples go beyond just this. If a woman had a conflicted relationship with her own mother, the label of "mom" may be complicated for her, and this may interfere with her ability to settle into this role. If a woman was frequently told how to act or what to do by her parents, this may make it difficult for her to feel empowered and make her own decisions about the care of her baby, and she may doubt that she really does know what is best. If a woman's own mother appeared as "selfless" and dedicated herself and everything that she had to her children, it might be difficult for this woman to give herself permission to take *her* needs into account when she has a baby of her own. For many women, the conflict of being both a daughter and a mother shows itself during visits "back home" when old patterns from childhood inevitably resurface and, suddenly, she becomes both a mother and someone else's child simultaneously.

How does this all show up in a mom's postpartum depression? Identity shifting is a huge part of the early weeks and months of parenthood, and all this old stuff can ignite feelings of anxiety, depression, anger, and can ignite feelings of anxiety, depression, and anger, leaving moms feeling overwhelmed. Those moms whose biochemistry is out of balance may have a hard time separating what is happening in the moment from what is being resurfaced. So these moms are likely to blame themselves and feel like they are failing at motherhood. Separating their own experience being parented from their experience parenting their own child can be a complicated project.

I had a mom and nine-month-old daughter in my office recently, and our conversation went as follows:

"I just can't bear to hear her cry," the mom says with tears in her eyes. "I am failing her. I can't get her what she needs, no matter how hard I try. She must hate me. I mean, she just looks at me with these eyes of desperation like she knows that I will always disappoint her."

I look at the new mom and her daughter, sitting on the sofa in front of me. Closely entwined. The baby's head rests delicately and sweetly on her shoulder, and she plays gently with her mama's long hair. This mom, instinctively, caresses the top of her head with her cheek. I can almost see them breathing together. This is not a baby whose needs aren't being met. This is without a doubt a baby who loves her mama deeply.

I ask her to consider whether this fear of hers feels familiar to her. If she has, at some point, been in a situation in which she can relate to how she imagines her baby girl must feel in the situation that she is envisioning.

The tears fall. "Yes," this mom says. "I am so afraid that she will feel the way that I felt as a kid."

And the work begins.

When Postpartum Depression Rises Up out of the Buried Traumas of Childhood

I was having dinner with a friend one night, and she shared with me some real concerns about someone she knew who had been extremely anxious since her now 2 ½ year-old daughter was born. Did this mom have postpartum depression? My friend described someone who had a nearly impossible time letting her daughter be apart from her. She held her constantly. She had yet to leave her child with anyone other than herself (meaning, of course, that she had not had a break in several years). She grew fearful anytime her kiddo cried, she panicked anytime her child needed something and she was unsure of what that particular thing was, and she was simply unable to tolerate any independence that this little girl was seeking. Let me also explain to you that this woman was also described as highly competent, loving, and social. This woman's anxiety and insecurities had, apparently, shown themselves only after her baby was born.

As is typical in these situations, this mama had become very isolated and hadn't connected much with other new moms. Her marriage was struggling. Family and friends were having a hard time managing their own frustrations with this mom's behaviors, no matter how much they wanted to help and support her. This mom was pushing everyone away, so it seemed, except for her daughter, whom she held close to her with a sort of apparent desperation.

I listened attentively as my friend described a situation that felt critical to her, and which she was confused by. Indeed, this sounded like a situation that was thick with layers of confusion and conflict for everyone involved. I had heard similar stories numerous times. I had never met the mom whom my friend was describing and so was in no place to fully assess the situation, but the themes and conflicts that this mom was experiencing were easy to identify. It was certainly possible that she had postpartum depression or anxiety.

As it turns out, this is a woman who was adopted at the age of two. Although she was raised by loving and attentive parents, she had always struggled with the uncertainty and feelings of ungroundedness that exist for many people who were adopted. This woman has no concrete memories of her earliest years, but as described by my friend, she had a clear sense of loss connected to this time. Yet, she had never discussed these feelings with anyone in depth and had not been in therapy at any point in her life. Until becoming a mom, she had, very successfully, managed her life in a way that allowed her to move through it with relative ease.

Then she became a mom and—WHAM—this ability seemed to falter.

Many, many women who have some early childhood experiences that are marked by early attachment challenges with their parents, trauma, childhood abuse, and/or conflict, and who feel that their earliest needs were not met, struggle with a fear around what it means to be apart from, separate from, or "unavailable" to their own children. These moms are terrified that their own kiddos will feel abandoned by them, that they will be unable to meet their every need, and that they will somehow let their babies down. And so, they may overcompensate. Often, these moms feel great fear and anxiety when apart from their little ones for even a moment. They don't give themselves permission to take breaks. They feel overwhelming anxiety when unable to soothe their babies' cries or when unable to read their cues and meet their needs. They are hard on themselves, and they set expectations for themselves as mothers that aren't humanly possible.

And this makes sense. These loving and dedicated moms want for their kids what they didn't have. The only challenge here is that they might not have a road map for how to do this in a way that is healthy for both themselves and their little ones. And, often, these moms may not be aware that the postpartum anxiety and/or postpartum depression that they feel is not just due to the challenges of the postpartum period but may also be due to very early experiences that are full of emotion that is hard to make sense of. When these moms don't reach out for support, their past and present experiences can become blurred and, despite attempts and desires to be thoughtful and proactive moms, they get into a pattern of parenting that is reactionary; they are, in effect, reacting to their own early experiences and are filled by great anxiety and emotional vulnerability in the process.

This is, to be clear, *not* the experience of every mom who was adopted herself. But postpartum depression is common for those who've experienced childhood trauma or abandonment. Working with a trained professional around these issues can be an important part of becoming the mom you want to be regardless of your own early childhood. Once the past and present are untangled, many of these moms feel a great sense of freedom, empowerment, and relief. And they find that they can settle into their role as Mom in a way that they never had imagined.

How Shame Gets in the Way of Postpartum Depression Recovery

Shame. It's a strong word, right?

Mental illness is associated with all kinds of stereotypes: *homelessness, joblessness, filth, insanity, murder, suicide, "craziness," inadequacy, incapability* ... so many words and images that are frightening and downright unacceptable to many, many people. These stereotypes are also inaccurate, although many people who don't have all the correct information may not think so. Because of the misinformation that exists about mental illnesses like postpartum depression and anxiety, people feel great shame when symptoms of mental illness become part of their reality. It's no longer something to discuss about "other" people, but something that is happening to themselves. When emotional suffering and mental illness happen after a new baby is born, at a time when the world leads us to believe that we are supposed to feel our best, shame can be at an all-time high.

"How can a good, loving, acceptable mother also be mentally ill?" so many ask. It just doesn't fit the picture that we hold of new mothers when we also associate this term with the above stereotypes, does it?

Mental illness is a term that can feel harsh and critical and unfamiliar to many moms who suffer. Yet, the definition of "mental illness" isn't as scary as we might assume. When I went online to see what definitions I could come up with, this is what I found:

Mental Illness:

1. *Any of various psychiatric conditions, usually characterized by impairment of an individual's normal cognitive, emotional, or behavioral functioning, and caused by physiological or psychosocial factors*
2. *Any of various disorders in which a person's thoughts, emotions, or behavior are so abnormal as to cause suffering to himself, herself, or other people*
3. *Any of various psychiatric disorders or diseases, usually characterized by impairment of thought, mood, or behavior*

"Impairment of thought, mood, or behavior" that is "abnormal" to that particular person. This is what it means to be mentally ill. To be depressed or anxious. To have postpartum depression, postpartum OCD, or postpartum PTSD. Truthfully, although not every new mom will suffer with depression or anxiety after having a baby, it is fair to say that nearly every mom will experience some impairment of thought, mood, or behavior when they suddenly enter motherhood. With depletions in sleep, nutrition, and support, this is almost inevitable to some degree.

But back to the impact of shame. This is what I have seen in my work with moms:

The mom who waits for 10 months to call for support and is, at this point, stuck in a myriad of symptoms that are debilitating.

The mom who is pulling out her hair (a condition known as trichotillomania) but who, despite a close relationship with her husband, will not let him know how deeply she struggles.

The mom who has tried everything to feel better—healthy nutrition, help at night so that she can sleep, childcare help so that she can take breaks and get exercise, reduced and more realistic expectations of herself as a mom—yet still suffers from extreme anxiety and depression but who will not try the medicine that is prescribed by her reproductive psychiatrist.

The mom who desperately needs community and love and support but who hides from those she cares about because she cannot bear the thought of them knowing that she is not okay.

I am telling you: Shame gets in the way of recovery and wellness.

Truthfully, this is a job for each of us. Every woman who has struggled with postpartum depression and who speaks openly about this begins that important job of reducing stigma. Every partner who nonjudgmentally supports a mother breaks this down just a little more. Every blog post, every authentic media effort, every mental health awareness day helps the public learn more. Every time a man or woman steps up and tells a story in an effort to inform, validate, and support, one more mother might gain the courage to step on shame's head.

Bam.

We need you.

When All You Want Is Out

Clinically, we call them *escapist fantasies*, but for many women, this term simply does not fit the bill. For many moms, these do not feel like fantasies; they are more like noble truths that cannot be debated.

"I can't do this."

"I want Out."

"This baby is better off without me."

"I think adoption is the best choice."

"I need to leave my marriage."

Often, no matter how hard someone tries to make this mama feel better—no matter how much someone else believes that she is the perfect mom for this baby and that she will get better—she sees no alternative.

It is a bit of a catch, you see. Hopelessness, despair, and lack of perspective are common symptoms of depression. This mom may feel as though the only way that she will feel better is if her life is different, when, really, it is often the depression or anxiety that is talking and once this mom *is* better, she will most likely feel differently about her situation and her life. But when smack in the middle of this emotionally painful place, this perspective is almost impossible to hold.

I saw a mom in my office once who was in this very place. I caught myself trying desperately to help her to experience hope and to understand that she is the perfect mom for her baby just the way she is, and that she will get better. Then I realized that this was not helping. What this mom needed more than anything else was to be seen, heard, and witnessed for the intensity of her pain, fear, and hopelessness.

THIS is what was real to her.

So, this chapter comes to all of you who can relate to the comments above. To all of you who feel, or have felt, that you cannot feel this way for one more day, hour, minute, or second. I hear you. It is an awful place to be, and I know that it feels intolerable to a degree that is inexplicable.

As I said to the mom in my office that day, perhaps there is room for both. Perhaps the place that you are in can feel debilitating and the only answer you can find is to get out. Now. Perhaps a different perspective is waiting for you. It is very possible that you can feel the way that you do now—in all its realness—and also feel differently soon. When support is obtained, when your biochemistry is normalized through medication if this is necessary, when your fears and anxieties and ambivalence are all addressed in therapy, you may want nothing more than to stay. Right where you are.

I am hopeful of this.

IV. SOCIAL HEALTH:
Your Relationships & Community

PPD and Attachment

Each woman who becomes a mother wants to have a solid, strong, and healthy attachment with her baby. With that, I think it's fair to assume, each mother fears on some level that this will not occur. Some moms worry that they won't have the tools to bond and attach appropriately because their own relationships with their parents are conflicted. Others fear that they won't be able to create an attachment as strong as the one they had with their own mom or dad. Others may find that their histories have contributed to a sort of "overcompensation" with their own kids, and they feel that the only way to attach is to give all of themselves. Some moms may feel that they don't have the knowledge or experience to attach appropriately with their little ones. Almost every mom who struggles with a mood and anxiety disorder like postpartum depression (PPD) worries about attachment. Attachment, it seems, is one of those hidden dilemmas that make early mothering feel overwhelming for most of us.

I want to talk a bit about what we know regarding healthy attachments between moms and babies. Please know that while I will be highlighting mom-baby attachment specifically, I also recognize how valuable and important dad and baby, second mom and baby, partner and baby, extended family and baby, and care provider and baby attachments are. In most situations, babies and children are fortunate to be loved and cared for by many individuals with whom their bonds are secure and valuable. And in most situations, it requires many caregivers to ensure that little people get what they need to thrive.

For the sake of this, let me give you two definitions:

1. *Attachment:* refers to the emotional connection that babies form with their caregivers. Attachments are built on shared experiences over time that contribute to a sense of trust and connection.
2. *Healthy attachment:* supports a child's social and emotional development throughout his or her life. Healthy attachments develop when a mom (or other primary caretaker) is able to respond to a baby's cues in a dependable way.

Moms who are depressed and/or anxious in the first few weeks, months, or years of motherhood get caught in a bind around forming healthy attachments. Often these moms feel immense guilt about not feeling well. They assume they will have difficulty attaching with their babies because of their PPD, and they overcompensate for this by feeling an even greater need to give all of themselves all the time (or, in some instances, stepping away entirely). This backfires. These moms, who believe that they need to be with their babies more to form strong attachments, become depleted and less able to be present and stay attuned to their baby's cues and needs. Then they feel more guilty and put more pressure on themselves to be available. Or they fear that their symptoms will destroy their little ones, and so they withdraw completely. Depression and anxiety complicate the already confusing picture around attachment and leave many women feeling unsure about what the relationship with their baby holds.

Here are a few things to keep in mind when it comes to healthy attachment:

1. For an attachment to be strong, a mom does not need to be with her baby all the time.

What matters most in a strong mom-baby attachment is the "quality" of time moms spend with their babies, and not the quantity. Babies thrive in relationships in which their caregivers can be present enough to validate their emotions, respond to both their emotional and physical needs, and understand the cues that suggest distress, need, contentment, and happiness. Sometimes a mom's perceived need to be with her baby all the time depletes her in a way that makes this kind of presence impossible. Being present all the time just isn't realistic. When babies feel that their moms are "seeing" them, even in small doses, their attachment and bond grows.

2. Mistakes are an important part of healthy attachments.

The idea that a mom needs to be perfect does not pan out when it comes to research. What helps build a strong attachment between mom and baby is mom's ability to acknowledge her own mistakes and to initiate what is called "repair" in the relationship. When a mom never makes a mistake, her baby (or child) misses out on the opportunity to learn about unconditional love, forgiveness, and being human. Strong bonds are not those that occur when mistakes are not made but are those that occur when mistakes are made and then repair of those mistakes follows. Moms who can acknowledge their shortcomings offer a key piece to relationship building.

3. Plenty of disappointment occurs in healthy attachments.

I cannot tell you how many times I work with women who are hugely worried about disappointing their children or making their children angry. These are often the moms who have a difficult time tolerating disappointment themselves and so worry that if they disappoint their own children, they will push them away. Again, what matters in strong attachments is that mom can acknowledge her inability to be perfect and that she can balance this (very human!) imperfection with an appropriate effort to make sure that her child's needs are met by someone else (remember, what matters in forming healthy attachment is that you can read and respond to your child's cues, not necessarily that you are the one to meet those needs all of the time). This example refers to the mom who has her partner put her baby to bed so that she can get out to see a friend or take a break, to the mom whose baby is in childcare so that she can work or take time for herself, and to the mom who is unable to breastfeed or chooses to formula-feed so that she can be well.

4. Responding appropriately to your baby's needs does not always mean that you will respond immediately.

As most of you probably know by now, it is not always possible to respond immediately to our baby's or children's needs. But, again, what matters in healthy attachment is that your kiddo feels that his or her need is being seen and recognized. Sometimes this response is not immediate. Sometimes you will need to acknowledge with your little one that you aren't able to meet a specific want (or need) in the moment. When moms can let their babies know that they hear them and understand that they need something, attachment is being formed even when this need is not met right away.

Often, moms set expectations of themselves that are based on misconceptions around attachment and that are insurmountable and unrealistic. Often, moms assume that to be attached to their babies (and for their babies to be attached to them), they need to, literally, be attached all of the time. Here are some examples that I see in my office:

- The mom who, despite her fatigue, growing impatience, and depletion, tells herself that she must be the one to feed her baby, put her baby to bed, and comfort her baby when he/she is distressed. This mom feels immense guilt when she is away from her baby, and yet feels disastrously tired when she is with her.
- The mom who feels pressure to continue breastfeeding her baby even when this process is making her physically or emotionally sick.
- The mom who feels uncontrollable anxiety around making mistakes or not getting it right the first time.

These moms fear that not being able to achieve the above is a determining factor in how attached they will be to their babies. Sound familiar?

So here is the deal, inspiring moms: Struggling with a postpartum mood or anxiety disorder like postpartum depression does not mean that you will not attach with your baby. But it does mean that without breaks, time to heal, rest, and support, giving your baby what he or she needs to form a healthy attachment with you will be difficult. To be dependable, to read your baby's cues, and to be consistent (we are focusing on quality, not quantity, remember...) you will need to reach out for support and begin the process of getting well. Sometimes this will mean stepping away. Or sharing the load with someone else. Or being less than perfect.

In helping to strengthen the healthy attachment with your baby, ask yourself the following:

- Can I let my baby know that I hear him even when I can't respond to his need right away?
- Do I have a sense of my baby's unique ways of communicating her needs?
- Can I spend at least one short, specific period each day looking into my baby's eyes, playing, and encouraging laughter?
- Can I bring in support when I notice that my baby has a need that I cannot meet?
- What do I need to do to take care of myself so that I can be as present and consistent with my baby as possible?

Finding Strength in Numbers During Postpartum Depression

Nobody talks about the isolation that creeps up in early motherhood. Before our babies are born, so many of us imagine lines of people wanting to come and visit our new little bundles. We also imagine wanting those people in our homes. We might assume that we will "live life as normal" and simply cart our little ones with us wherever we might want to go. We imagine that we will want to go places. We have daydreams about getting together with our friends who also have little ones, just to gab about how wonderful motherhood is. And we also imagine that motherhood will be wonderful all the time.

However, once those babies are born, many moms—especially those who are suffering from a postpartum mood disorder like postpartum depression—find that they don't want to engage in any of these previously mentioned activities, or they find they don't have the energy to tackle the mountain of logistics that are needed just to get out the door. If moms finally do manage to get to a place where they are in the company of others, many fear most of all that the people around them will see that they aren't living all their earlier fantasies and that in reality, well, they just aren't happy.

Many moms spend countless hours alone with their babies, wondering if they are doing anything right. Worrying about milk quantities, sleep position, reflux, and fussiness. They suffer alone in their world of frightening anxieties and uncertainties. Many of these moms get so used to their anxiety and their isolation that they begin to wonder if it is just part of what it means to be a new mom. And when someone mentions a new moms group? Well, for most of these moms, it's the *last thing* they want to do. For moms who are suffering with postpartum depression, being around other moms who are assumed to be having an easy time or who feel the need to talk at length about how incredible motherhood is feels like being sent straight to the boiler room.

But here is the thing: We know that groups, be they support groups, community groups, therapy groups, or mom and baby groups, are a really important part of the recovery process for many women who are suffering. When facilitated appropriately, getting together with other women who are feeling as isolated, anxious, overwhelmed, conflicted, powerless, lost, and exhausted as you can provide unmatched validation, support, education, and encouragement. Groups of women offer the chance to truly express one's voice, to practice being real, and to share strategies, successes, and disappointments with others who get what you are going through. Perhaps often most healing is that chance to be in a group with those who, on the outside, you might assume have it all together but who are sitting right next to you with the same worries.

Your baby might benefit too. A study conducted at the Shanghai International

Peace Maternity and Child Health Hospital (now, how's that for a name!) has determined that maternal group psychotherapy not only reduces the risk of postpartum depression for moms but also has an impact on the temperament of their babies. Moms who attended a six-week psychotherapy group focusing on prenatal and postpartum depression and anxiety and the risk factors for these conditions reported a higher level of easy infant temperament than mothers in a control group. So, the group resulted in not just happier moms, but also happier babies (or at least the moms felt that way)!

So, I encourage you...give it a go. Postpartum Support International has coordinators in every state, many of whom have set up support groups for moms like you or know where the local ones are. If you can't find one, there is always the option of finding a trained professional to help you start one yourself. If you have already begun to tell your story, you've probably noticed that once you open your mouth, others chime in and share their stories too. Strength in numbers, my friends. You are all part of one great army of Warrior Moms.

Keeping Your Relationship on Track During Postpartum Depression

We know that marital and relationship conflict is a risk factor for developing postpartum depression. We also know that perinatal mood and anxiety disorders (PMADs) can cause great distress in marriages and relationships. It is a bit of the "what comes first" debate, and on one hand, it doesn't matter much. What does matter is that partners find a way to appreciate and support each other during this time so that both of their needs are met, and so that the baby's needs are met too.

Research has shown us that while partners who report *satisfaction* in their marriages are more likely to also report positive attitudes toward their infants and their roles as parents, partners who report *dissatisfaction* in their marriages are more likely to spend less time bonding and attaching with their babies. This is especially true for dads who, when in conflict with their spouses, are likely to pull away from both mom and their little one.

So, with all of this said, I offer some suggestions for getting back on track.

Please note that these are only suggestions and that really making some of this stuff happen often requires outside support from a trained therapist. (See the Resources section for help in locating a therapist in your area.) If you are already in therapy for treatment of postpartum depression or anxiety, or antenatal depression or anxiety, and haven't already, inviting your spouse or partner to a session or two so that he/she can become aware of how to best support you might be a great start.

1. Never assume that your spouse/partner knows what you need. I know that this can be really frustrating, but I swear to you, waiting for him/her to read your mind will keep you waiting forever. This is not fair to either of you.
2. Become as clear as you can possibly be on what your needs are right now before you attempt to communicate them to someone else. This can be hard to figure out, so outside help can be really useful.
3. Realize that your partner is probably scared and overwhelmed too and that he/she is also going through a giant transition. Many, many dads and non-birth moms whose wives/partners are depressed become depressed as well. It is important that you both receive the support you need.
4. Carve out quality time to talk. Yes, I know this one isn't easy either, but it is hugely important. If you haven't already, spend time talking about your hopes, joys, fears, anxieties, and uncertainties about parenting. Highlight the places where you agree and see if you can negotiate where you don't. Understand as best you can that you will each bring your own experiences into your choices and instincts around parenting. This is often where past

and present blend, and your relationship together thus far may be primarily based on what you know about each other as adults.

5. Find ways, together, to invent yourselves as parenting partners. It is very common for couples to feel as though they have two very different relationships: one when they are parenting their children (with all the logistics) and one when they are on their own during couple time.
6. The relationships that report greatest satisfaction are those that can be described as "close" and "confiding." There are a million ways to exemplify this, and each relationship will be unique. But having the goal—together—of working in this direction is golden. In what ways can you feel more "close"? Can you spend more time telling each other that you love each other? Can you hold each other when going to bed at night? Can you leave notes for each other? Can you hold hands more? Schedule in time to be intimate? Can you make sure you each get a hug a day? **How can you be more "confiding"?** How can you communicate more directly with each other? How can you make sure that each of you is able to express your needs from the other?

Taking care of yourself is such an important part of taking care of your babies... and this goes for taking care of the relationship with your spouse/partner as well.

This can be hard work, folks, I know. But man, oh man, does the hard work pay off. If you and your partner are having difficulty doing this hard work on your own (and this is difficult for most), outside help might be the key. Chances are that with a more solid relationship, your recovery from PPD will feel easier.

How Postpartum Depression Affects Your Marriage or Partnership

While we know that the first year after having a baby is statistically the most difficult for marriages and partnerships, we certainly cannot say that every woman who is struggling with postpartum depression or a related illness will also be in a marriage or partnership full of conflict. Nor can we say that women who are in conflicted relationships are also all working their way through perinatal mood and anxiety disorders.

However, I am pretty sure that most of us in partnerships who have given birth to or adopted babies can agree that major shifts happen in relationships at home that require a significant amount of work, understanding, and reinventing. We know that inadequate social support, including marital conflict, is one of the risk factors in the development of postpartum depression and/or anxiety.

So, with that said, let's talk about sex. Well, not entirely, but let's talk about relationships and the often emotionally challenging shifts and changes that occur when a baby enters the picture. Research has identified five major changes that couples go through when they become parents, and each of these changes can lead to conflict between partners:

1. Regardless of the choices that couples have made prior to becoming parents, gender roles become more traditional once a baby is born. Caring for an infant can add 30 to 50 hours of additional "work" a week for parents, and it is common for women to take on two to three times more of these parenting responsibilities than men, regardless of whether they are working inside or outside of the home.
2. Once a baby is born, significantly less time exists for uninterrupted couple-focused communicating.
3. Often, when a new baby joins a family, disposable income declines due to the new financial responsibilities that come along with that new bundle. This will often mean fewer individual and shared leisure activities (which often means less individual and couple self-care time).
4. Parenting is a busy time. Once a baby enters the picture, frequency and quality of couple time is significantly reduced.
5. For most couples, intimacy and the frequency of intercourse change for months after having a baby. After delivery, many women feel discomfort and/or pain with intercourse, and most couples are exhausted after sleepless days and nights of caring for a newborn. Combine that with the demands of breastfeeding for those who go this route, and many couples will spend much less time being intimate. In fact, one study showed that 50 percent of

women and 20 percent of men report reduced sexual responsiveness for 6 to 12 months postpartum. One-third of couples will report this reduced sexual responsiveness two to three years after birth. Women who are struggling with depression will have an extra challenge here as lowered libido is one of the very common symptoms of depression and at times a side effect of anti-depressant medication.

So, what does all this mean? What this means is that having a baby is HARD on a marriage or partnership. Add postpartum depression and other mood disorders, and this relationship stuff becomes even harder.

In the work that I do with moms who are struggling with perinatal mood and anxiety disorders, the following issues come up around marriages and relationships:

1. Many women are skilled at hiding the true nature of their emotional vulnerability. Often husbands and partners do not know how much they are really struggling.
2. Despite this, most women expect (or wish?) that their husbands and partners will know what to do to support them.
3. Many of these women are very reluctant to ask for help for fear they will disappoint, scare, or push away their partners.
4. When depressed, many moms will retreat into social isolation and withdrawal. This is often confusing for partners, as mom will often pull away from him/her as well.
5. Dads usually expect moms to be joyful in early parenting, and so they are often unprepared for the unexpected challenges if a mom becomes depressed or anxious. Dads may need to take on more nurturing and household chores than they were expecting, and moms may feel incredible guilt over this.
6. Partners might know each other well as individuals, but do not necessarily know each other as parents yet. Both mom and non-birth mom/dad can become disappointed, angry, fearful, and confused when these new identities develop if they are not what they each expected. If mom is suffering with a mood disorder, her partner can suddenly become overwhelmed with questions about where his wife/partner "went"—and of course, mom is wondering the same thing. This may be the first time that dad has witnessed his/her partner in such distress.
7. Most women will express feelings of disappointment, resentment, anger, and/or sadness around the ways that their partners are reacting to the changes that occur with a new baby. Most of these women will also be at a loss as to what to do with these feelings. And many of these women will feel as though their relationships are doomed.

Talking with someone trained to support couples through the transition to parenthood can be incredibly empowering and connecting. The strongest couples I know are those who have participated in some sort of counseling support. We don't know what we don't know. Learning about each other in the process of becoming a parent is an important way to move forward on this journey together.

Postpartum Depression and Relationships: Treating the Whole Family

Moms who suffer with postpartum depression and anxiety feel alone. Almost always. They feel misunderstood, unseen, isolated, and lost. When they sit in my office, moms who suffer with a perinatal mood or anxiety disorder tell me they feel like they are in battle all by themselves.

But here is the thing, and perhaps one of the biggest differences between treating postpartum depression and treating generalized depression and anxiety: The moms who sit in my office are not my *only* clients. When I treat a mom for symptoms of depression and anxiety, I am also treating the whole family. She exists within the context of all her relationships: the one with her baby, her other children, her husband/partner, her own parents, her friends, and her extended community. I cannot treat that mom for her symptoms without understanding the deep complexity between her symptoms and the rest of her world. Postpartum depression/anxiety is one big tangle of symptoms and relationships, and to work with that mom in a bubble simply misses the most complex piece of these challenges: She is suffering at a time when relationships matter *most.*

One mom feels detached from her baby and worries that she will never love him as she should. One mom loves her baby so much that she is afraid to ever let her cry or be cared for by others. One mom's pregnancy was unwanted or unplanned, and she feels resentment for the growing belly or the baby whom she wants desperately to love but feels anger toward. One mom feels unable to manage her toddler once the new baby comes or feels unrelenting guilt about not being able to give enough of herself to anyone. One mom feels let down by her partner and wants nothing more than to be understood by the person she knows best. One mother feels a new wave of anger toward her own parents for not providing her with what she feels she needed during her own childhood or for not being there to support her now, as she suffers. One mom feels threatened by her in-laws, and her uncertainty around these relationships is interfering with her marriage. One mom feels let down by her community of friends during a time when she needs them so much. For each of these moms, recovery comes not just in the reduction of symptoms, but also in the repair of the relationships that feel so damaged to her.

So how do I do this? Attention is paid to her definition of a "good enough mother," her development of confidence with her baby, and work around attachment and bonding. We invite dads and partners in to discuss missed communication, each other's needs and expectations, and ways to work together as a team to get mom (and her family) well. We talk of new boundaries and shifting relationships with parents and in-laws so that mothers feel comfortable with the changes that occur in these relationships when a baby is born. We do work around asking for and receiving support from community so that she feels more connected and less alone. We talk with those people who are important to her (partners, parents, friends, siblings, in-laws) about what postpartum depression and related illnesses are so that the judgment decreases, and the understanding and support become more tangible.

You have heard it before: *Happy mom, happy family*. At times, this statement may feel like an undue amount of pressure that is put on a mother to be well for others. The way I see it, mom and family are so interrelated during postpartum depression that the many players deserve support and attention in the effort to get mom well. She cannot do it all alone, nor should she be expected to.

So, moms, if you are suffering and feel alone, know that you are not. Others need you as much as you need them even if these are relationships that may need readjusting and repair. When you sit in my office, or the office of any other expert in postpartum depression, know that you are being seen both as an individual and as a part of something much larger than you, even if you may not feel connected to much of anything at the moment.

Postpartum Depression: When Dads and Partners Don't Seem to Get It

You are struggling—*really* struggling—and all you want (besides symptom relief) is for your partner to get it—for your partner to truly empathize, for him or her to take you in his or her arms and just be there with you during postpartum depression.

You want a gaze of understanding, a hand to reach to, and an unconditional smile that lets you know that this person is right alongside you through your pain and suffering, no matter what. But sometimes, dads and partners don't seem to get it, do they?

Certainly, partners like this exist (they are usually the ones who call my office looking for the support their families need), but often this picture looks very different. Often, what it *feels* like to struggling moms is this: *They just don't get it! They keep telling me that I should be happy because we have such a beautiful baby! They get to go to work, see friends, talk about other things than poop and spit-up, and get to the gym, and they say that they're tired! Why are they getting on me for the house being dirty? Why do they keep trying to have sex? Don't they get it that I have nothing else to give? Why do they keep giving me that look that makes me feel like such a failure?*

On the other hand, here's what the second parent may be feeling: *"I just can't do enough! What does she want from me? Why can't she be happy like we talked about? What is happening? Why isn't this parenting thing what we expected? Why am I so angry all the time? She has no energy for me anymore! Why does she keep looking at me like I am such a failure?"*

We know, through all of the research and firsthand reports, that moms with postpartum depression and related illnesses who feel supported at home get well quicker than those who do not. What this means is that second parents and partners play a tremendous role in a mom's recovery...whether they know it or not.

We also know that becoming a new parent is not a cakewalk for dads and non-birth moms either. Up to 10 percent of dads and non-birth moms will suffer from an episode of postpartum depression or anxiety, and, often, these second parents struggle quietly, or they become irritated and angry, isolated and withdrawn, or blaming. We know dads and non-birth moms often feel as scared as moms by the unexpected realities of new parenthood. We know they want to be useful but don't know how to be. We know they miss you as much as *you* miss you. We know they go through identity changes as well, become anxious about the "what ifs," and miss their old lives and friends and ability to feel free of responsibility just like you do. We know they bring their own unresolved issues from their upbringing with them when they become parents, too. In other words, we know that moms and dads are not as separate in their experiences as it often feels to them.

And so, what happens at home? Mom suffers, and dad suffers, and they do so independently of one another. Mom gets resentful of dad, and dad gets resentful of mom. There is a lot of pressure to mind read. Mom feels that dad should know what to do to support her through postpartum depression, and dad feels that mom should appreciate his efforts at work and at home when he tries to fix things. Both mom and dad begin to feel swallowed up in the unknown, in the lost familiarity, and in the frustration of "not being able to do enough." Because they feel that they can't support the other in the way they desire, they stop trying. They become distant. They muddle through until the straw breaks the camel's back and someone says something they later wish they hadn't. Or worse.

Whenever possible, I request that dads and partners accompany moms to their sessions in my office. I encourage that she brings her partner along for at least one or two sessions in the beginning so that her partner can gain some perspective and the two of them can discuss a plan for support at home. I don't require this, but when it happens, it is hugely helpful.

Often moms and dads take me up on this offer (such a symbol of caring and effort!), and when this happens, the increase in feelings of closeness is usually visceral; I can feel it begin to take hold in my office. Sometimes this is not the case, of course. Sometimes dynamics make it difficult for dad to meet mom where she is; sometimes cultural differences play a role, sometimes longer-standing issues in a partnership really need some work to begin to untangle, and sometimes deep shame and stigma around mental illness make it challenging for dads and partners to truly hear what is happening and to acknowledge their part in recovery. However, creating an opportunity for partners to slow down and really look at what is happening is a very important first step in family recovery. It can take the blame off of each individual and bring the responsibility for support and recovery back to the team.

Dads and partners *do* want to help you to get well. But here's the catch, moms: They cannot do this alone. They need *your* help to be able to help *you*. They want to know what to "do" and how to be. Invite them to a therapy session if you haven't already. Sit down and try to find the places where you can relate to each other. (Do you *both* feel angry, scared, overwhelmed, or frustrated?) What do you want to ask of him or her to support you? (Help with the baby? More understanding about household chores? More awareness about postpartum depression? More patience? More "I love you's"?) What does he or she need from you to be able to give this of himself or herself? (More understanding of his experience? Exercise? Information?) In other words, neither of you can do this alone. You need each other, and with each other, you will see the light at the end of the tunnel calling to you much more quickly.

You need each other to get through postpartum depression.

And your babies and children need both of you.

For simplicity in this chapter, I have often used the words "dad" and "he." Please know, however, that I acknowledge the diversity of families, and at any point "partner" and "she" can be substituted.

For more stories that may help dads understand postpartum depression and how to help you through it, see the Resources section.

When Relationships Worsen After Mothers Recover from Postpartum Depression

The women I see in my office constantly amaze me. These women work hard. They ask themselves difficult questions and do their best to uncover the answers that resonate most for them. They face their fears head-on. They exemplify a braveness that comes from a desire to get well. And they do.

So often, the women who leave my office for the last time after months of suffering, hard work, and recovery do so with a new sense of self that feels stronger, clearer, and more deserving than before postpartum depression or anxiety walked, uninvited, through their doors. Many of these women will continue to work with a therapist throughout their lifetime. Yet, even for these women, their suffering decreases or no longer exists when the crisis phase of their work is over.

This new self feels hopeful, and optimistic, and at ease. For many of them. For these women, now it is time to celebrate, time to realize that being a mom feels more "right" than "wrong." Time to celebrate a sky that looks bluer. Time to get to know a sense of self that feels more forgiving and human. And a time to (dare we say it?) be happy.

Yet, sometimes I see some of these moms back again only weeks after leaving my office for that final session. Understand, these moms are not back because their postpartum depression symptoms have returned so soon after they realized they were feeling better, although this is something almost every mom fears. These women are back because something unexpected has resulted from their new, emerging self: Their relationships with their partners have seemed to unravel.

It is a particular type of unraveling, one that feels different from when they were in the depths of postpartum depression despair. This type of marital/partner conflict seems to come out of recovery at a time when these moms finally feel their best. Rather than partner conflict coming at a time when these women feel incapable, it is coming at a time when they feel, perhaps, more capable than they ever have before.

Why is this? Why is it that just when a mom feels happier, better about herself, and more optimistic, she feels unable to connect with the person with whom she is the most intimate? Why is it that as she begins to feel more at ease, her relationship begins to feel even more difficult?

I have heard women say that their spouses/partners make the following statements:

"You have gotten better, but you have left me behind!"

"I thought things would be better between us when you got well, but now you seem

even more unhappy with me!"

"Why can't things just be the way they were before postpartum depression?"

Individual change is both exciting and strange, especially when it happens in the context of a relationship. When a mom recovers from a postpartum mood or anxiety disorder like postpartum depression, she often feels evolved somehow. She has learned limitless things about herself, including both who she wants to be and what she needs to feel her best.

While PPD may have been an unwelcome and unbelievably traumatic experience, the recovery process can allow for new insights that may have never been uncovered had it not been for the need for exploration. And, while these moms might have grown and changed through this process, their partners may not have. Because of this, suddenly, the dynamics of their relationships are different.

Postpartum mood and anxiety disorders change women. Thankfully, once they have recovered, a large number of these women will say that they have grown from their experiences and changed for the better; the necessity to slow down and explore the pieces that may have contributed to despair (be it lacking self-care or awareness about what is needed to feel her best, early childhood or family of origin issues, negative thought patterns and challenging belief systems, or undiagnosed and not yet treated mental illness) has actually created opportunity to grow. Man, oh man, do these women grow.

So, when a partner makes a comment like *"Why can't things be like they were before PPD?"* a new ripple of disconnect can be felt. *Before postpartum depression?* Very little remains the same after a woman experiences a postpartum mood or anxiety disorder. Relationships really do have to adjust to these changes. It is important to realize that while you may feel like a new and different person, your partner may not—and he or she may simply expect things to go back to "normal" and back to the way they were before the two of you negotiated this very turbulent journey.

Some couples may not make it through this journey. Statistics tell us that the first year after having a baby is often the most difficult in a couple's lifetime. Add postpartum depression into this already chaotic time, and the strength of a partnership may be too tested to remain intact.

However, before you decide that the two of you are incapable of weathering this storm or that your partner and relationship are unable to change with you, I encourage you to reach out for support from a trained couples therapist, from a spiritual counselor, or from someone else who has the skill and insight to walk you through the particulars of this new challenge, of the struggles and accomplishments of your past, and of the expectations and hopes for moving forward.

You might just find that your relationship is as capable as you are.

Love in the Time of Postpartum Depression

Is it possible to love your baby and simply *not* love the logistics that go into having a newborn? Yes. Yes. And yes.

This is, perhaps, the myth that is most voiced and debunked early on in my work with new moms. Moms who are struggling with postpartum depression feel so much guilt for not being well. They judge themselves up and down and around the block for dreading the nighttime feedings, for questioning whether or not they "should have done this," for feeling claustrophobic when holding their babies all day, for not enjoying breastfeeding, and for wanting—more than anything—a full night's sleep. Each mom who comes to see me for support postpartum is afraid, at least initially, that I will think she is not cut out for motherhood and that she is a "bad mom" for not loving the early weeks and months to pieces.

It is so easy for each of these moms to assume that they are the only ones who feel frustrated and (yes, I will say it) often *devastated* by the new responsibilities and life changes that come with being a parent. Yet, truly, most moms do feel this way at some point. In fact, several experts have described childbearing and becoming a mother as a *psychic trauma,* and *an existential crisis*. I mean, this shock to the system is real for almost everyone, and it is especially severe for those women who are struggling with postpartum depression or anxiety.

No matter how much they love their little ones.

So, try this on for size: **You can absolutely love your little nugget to pieces and not love *being* a mom right now.** You don't have to love changing diapers at 2 a.m., muddling through the often-unpleasant trials and errors of breastfeeding, and bouncing your baby at all hours of the night. You don't have to feel appreciative every moment that your baby fusses, or cries, or screams for the umpteenth hour in a row. You are allowed to wonder why the heck you did this. You are more than welcome to wish you were on a peaceful tropical island far away from all your responsibilities. You are allowed, most certainly, to be afraid and to wonder how on Earth such a little being has the power to control the lives of one or more competent and well-meaning adults. You don't have to know what to do, or how to soothe, or which baby-rearing books to believe. None of these things cancel out your love for your baby. None of them. Moms who are struggling postpartum love their children just as much as those who are not.

I know that I am preaching to the choir here.

But still, no matter how much the moms in my office know within themselves that they love their babies, they still wonder if others will doubt this. It is a sort of *either-or* mix-up. As if the rule stated that you *either* love your baby and everything about being a mother, *or* you don't love motherhood and therefore must not love your baby. How unfair and inaccurate this is!

So, my friends, I am hopeful that you can be kind to yourselves and allow a bit of fairness back into your perception of what you are going through. You get to choose whether or not early motherhood resonates for you, and, even if it does not, you can be thankful for that baby who rests (or cries) in your arms.

Love most certainly DOES exist in the time of postpartum depression.

Is Someone Holding Your Postpartum Depression Against You?

Postpartum depression changes you. No doubt about it. It can also change your partner, children, extended family, and friends. Thankfully and for the most part, these changes are positive ones—although it is certainly difficult to see this side of things when you are smack in the middle of your recovery. But I can say with complete honesty that when moms have received adequate support during their illness, more times than not, women and families leave behind their postpartum mood and anxiety disorders feeling a greater sense of self, a greater ability to communicate their needs, and more prepared to keep themselves healthy and teach their little ones to do the same. I know that it is hard to hear when you are amidst the suffering, but postpartum depression can create opportunities for growth that women never saw coming.

Unfortunately, sometimes this is not the case. Sometimes a mom's diagnosis of postpartum depression and anxiety can be used against her in ways that can create feelings of entrapment, disgrace, and continued shame.

I have worked with these women in my office, and we have all heard about these moms in the media: These are the moms who can't seem to shake the label of "postpartum depressed," whatever they do. They are judged by partners, family members, friends, and, at times, society as a whole no matter how distant their diagnosis may be. Courts try to use their diagnoses against them in custody battles. Partners at home assume for years that any time they react emotionally to something, they are doing so because they have or had a postpartum mood or anxiety disorder. Family members and friends suddenly hold lesser expectations for success simply because these moms have at one time been unable to perform at their capacities. These women feel like they are taken less seriously. They feel less trusted. Their postpartum depression suddenly defines these moms in a way that does not allow them to be who they truly are outside of the illness they suffered from.

This can be unbearably frustrating, especially because you and I both know that PPD is an illness that does not define us. It is an illness that is treatable. It is an illness that does not equate to being a "bad" mother, not loving children, or being less of a woman. You and I both know that PPD does *not* mean that we are flawed and only means that our brains, bodies, and identities have shifted because of the inevitable biological, social, and psychological changes that occur with childbirth and becoming a mother. You and I both know that postpartum mood and anxiety disorders are not our fault.

It is important to realize that sometimes your fear of being judged, misunderstood, and misrepresented may be more real than the ways in which your illness is being held against you. This fear is a real thing, and almost every woman who suffers postpartum will hold some of this fear at least initially. *What if people think less of me? What if people assume that I am a bad mother because I am suffering? What if I completely lose myself? What if I am flawed?* Remember, my friends, simply because we think these things are true doesn't mean they are, and often it is us who hold these judgments and not necessarily those around us.

So, what do you do if you feel like you are being shoved in a box because of your illness? How can you begin the process of setting yourself free from the labels and judgments that sometimes tag along for years after you recover?

- Keep going to therapy. *Keep. Going. To. Therapy.* When feeling alone and misunderstood, it is hugely important to have at least one person who understands you, who can help you to see the bigger picture, and who can assist in the process of clarifying what is required to live the kind of life that is important to you. It is hugely unfair and unrealistic to assume that you should fight the fight all alone.
- Know the facts: Having a postpartum mood or anxiety disorder like postpartum depression is not a reason to take away custody in a court of law. It just isn't. In custody battles, a court will take many things into account, and a willingness to identify struggle, seek help, and make the efforts to get well will be one of these things. Having had postpartum depression does not make someone an unfit mother.
- Educate others. I know that this can feel exhausting, but usually people who are holding judgment are not adequately informed. Your partner, family, friends, and community may need some information around the facts, and sometimes you may be the only one who can provide this.
- Remember that reaching out for help when you are struggling is a big whopping strength and *not* a weakness. It takes guts to be vulnerable, admit to your struggles, and trust someone to help you through. This is a brave thing to do and in no way makes you someone who is weak, incapable, or flawed.
- Do your research. If you are struggling and are reaching out for help, do what you can to work with someone who is educated in the unique specifics of perinatal mood and anxiety disorders or who is willing to learn. It is important that you are able to trust that your therapist is not going to overreact to your struggles, is going to be able to educate you on all of the appropriate facts, and is, when appropriate, willing and able to include your partner or other important people in your recovery process. It is challenging to be vulnerable in therapy and important that when you are willing to do so, you know that you will be treated with respect and perspective.

- Find ways to trust yourself. Yes, finding ways to trust that you are bigger than your illness is imperative in the recovery process. Women who continue to judge themselves, who continue to feel flawed, and who are unable to connect with the strength that comes with having struggled postpartum (no matter how teeny tiny that feeling of strength may be) are more likely to put that out to others. Unintentionally, of course. But if you want others to believe in your capability and strength, you are going to need to believe in it yourself.

WHAT WE NEED TO LEARN FROM WOLVES

Wolves have a lot to teach us, people. Seriously.

Fact: Wolves travel in packs. When a female wolf gives birth to her pups, the entire wolf pack pitches in to care for both the mother and her young. When the mother wolf is still tired from birth, the *entire* pack hunts for her and her pups, bringing back food to feed the mama and her newborns. When mama wolf is strong enough to engage with the others, a "babysitter" wolf takes over with the pups so that she can take breaks to hunt, roam, and rest.

I am not making this stuff up.

So…when you are home with your baby, feeling as though you should be doing it all gracefully with no help from others, think of the wolves. I think they are on to something. They seem to know more than we do about community, self-care, and what's required for postpartum health.

V. GRIEF AND LOSS:
Baby Loss & Loss of Self

The Overlap between Miscarriage, Perinatal Loss, and PPD: 13 Things to Know about Grief

Losing a baby through miscarriage, elective termination, stillbirth, childbirth, after a NICU stay, sudden infant death syndrome (SIDS), or at any other time is, without a doubt, one of the most difficult experiences a parent will ever endure. A parent goes through unexplainable depths of despair when attempting to understand the shift that occurs when all hopes and expectations suddenly drop out from underneath anything stable.

It is an experience that many will never need to make sense of and also one that many others will swim through unexpectedly. It is tragic and drastic and totally and completely unfair, and yet thousands upon thousands of families find themselves in this position each year. Here is what we know:

- Approximately 15 to 20 percent of confirmed pregnancies end in miscarriage.
- In the US, the rate of stillbirth is documented as one in 160 to 200 pregnancies.
- In the US, SIDS affects between 5,000 to 7,000 infants every year.
- In the US, approximately 11,300 infants die within 24 hours of their birth each year.

I give these statistics not to scare you, but because it is important for those mothers who have lost their children to know that they are not alone and that many others like them are needing to navigate this loss, too.

I have worked with countless women in my office as they try to manage the unfamiliar emotions that surround loss, and I have learned a great deal from these phenomenal moms. I also have a dear friend and colleague who lost her daughter hours after birth, and she, too, has honored me with her insight, pain, and eventual healing.

With the information gathered from both my clients and my dear friend (who is now a clinician in San Francisco specializing in perinatal loss), this chapter is written for all of the moms who are trying to navigate the unfamiliar postpartum experience while also grieving the loss of a child who never made it home or past that first-year mark. For these moms, postpartum distress is complicated by the process of grief, and sometimes it is hard to make sense of what goes where in this unimaginable puzzle.

So, if you are one of these women, here is what I want you to know:

1. Some women who lose babies through miscarriage are able to move through this loss freely, while others feel deep despair at this loss. This process involves no "shoulds." There is no right way to feel. If you feel strong and grounded and ready to move forward after a miscarriage, that is totally valid. If you feel deep loss and grief, then that, too, is appropriate. No one gets to tell you how you feel except you.

2. Any time a body goes from being pregnant to not being pregnant, there is an important shift in hormones that significantly affects brain chemistry. Postpartum depression, anxiety, and other mood disorders can affect a mom regardless of the point at which a baby is delivered. You are likely in a position where you need to process through grief while also having a vulnerable brain chemistry. This can make the experience of healing feel impossible for many.

3. Grief is a normal process and includes a shifting of emotions such as denial, anger, bargaining, depression, and acceptance. Grief felt after the loss of a baby from miscarriage or other event is not necessarily depression, and despite overlap, it should not be treated as such. If you feel angry one day and dissociated from your loss the next, this is normal.

4. If you are not aware of a shifting through the stages of grief and continue to feel debilitated by your suffering, clinical depression or anxiety may need to be addressed. "Healthy" grief moves, but sometimes it can develop into relentless depression that requires more specific treatment. Many moms will experience depression that includes feelings of guilt, shame, self-doubt,

and sometimes suicidal ideation. Regaining a sense of self, hope, and trust is important to one's healing after a loss such as this.

5. Identity shifting is a huge piece of the postpartum experience for every new parent, and yet moms who lose their babies are not able to show the world their mother-ness. If you feel like a mom, and yet are not able to participate in the experiences that the mothers around you are included in, know that this is a shared experience and that, whether or not the world can see this, we value you as a mother too.
6. Loss can often beget feelings of loss. Many women who lose their babies become suddenly afraid of losing everything else, be it their sanity, other relationships important to them, their faith in the world, or any hope for the future. Many, many women who go through this loss feel a deep need to grab onto other things in their life for fear of losing those, too. If this is happening to you, let those close to you know.
7. Relationships with your spouse/partner, family, and friends will be impacted by your loss. It is important to be aware of the tendency to isolate during this time. Receiving appropriate support will be imperative in your healing, and you may have work to do in relearning your relationships given this new reality. If you are unable to get the support that you need from loved ones, reach out to a therapist who can help.
8. While you desperately want your spouse/partner to understand what you are going through, he/she may not. People grieve differently. Often, losing a baby is a very different experience for a mother than it is for her partner, as she was the one who felt the development of this baby and feels, still, the physical loss as her body adjusts to no longer being pregnant. Give space for your own process as well as your partner's.
9. You are likely to learn who your truest friends are during this time. Some people's insecurities and fears around loss and tragedy may interfere with their ability to be available to you. It is entirely appropriate for you to spend time with those who are able to give you what you need, and to take distance from those who are not.
10. It is normal to feel triggered into sadness and despair when you least expect it. You may find reminders in the places where you least intend them to be. Holidays and anniversaries as well as seeing pregnant women, babies, playgrounds, doctor's offices, and advertisements for baby-related items all may bring you to tears even when you feel strong. This is normal.
11. People don't always know what to say. You might want desperately to talk about your baby, to bring him or her to life through your words and

memories, to make room for your baby in conversation and in your experiences. Some people will worry that bringing up your baby and your loss in conversation will be upsetting to you. It is helpful to let the people in your life know what you need.

12. Just because you are ready to feel whole again, are healing, and may decide to have more children, this does not mean that the baby you lost is forgotten. Regaining strength does not mean that you have "moved on" and will no longer think of what might have been. Your pregnancy and your baby will always be a part of you. However, you deserve to be well, and the feeling that you must keep grieving in order to stay faithful to your baby will not serve you. Finding a way to honor your pregnancy or your baby through ritual or event is often a lovely way of incorporating that being into your life as you move forward.
13. Finally, find others who have experienced something similar. As mentioned, so many times in this book, community is imperative, and I am certain that others can offer you the kind of solace, strength, and integrity you will need as you continue to heal.

Having a Baby after Infant Loss: The Complicated Mix of Grief and Joy

The process of attempting to make sense of neonatal or infant loss is complicated and layered, and it leaves most women with uncertain and raw emotion that is not easily understood. I work with many women through their grief and eventual healing once a baby has passed, and while these women would give anything to have their babies with them in the ways that they had dreamed, they are usually aware and accepting of their own need for support during this impossibly difficult time.

But what about those women who go on to have healthy babies after losing a child? Are they finally happy and content and able to "move on" now that they have brought their babies home? Many people think this *should* be so ... but in reality, a large number of these women are hit hard with a depression or anxiety that is unwanted, unwelcome, and unexpected when the new baby arrives. And because these emotions are occurring at a time when these women want so desperately to be happy and connected to their babies, feelings of guilt, shame, and insecurity abound.

Each woman's experience is unique, and conflict can appear in many different ways:

- One mom is pregnant again or carries her newborn and must negotiate the all-too-frequent question of "Is this your first?"
- One mom looks at her baby for the first time and feels "nothing."
- One mom wants to feel joy as her new baby rolls over for the first time, but finds that she cannot.
- One mom's new baby is a boy, but secretly she is disappointed that he is not a girl like the baby she lost.
- One mom is riddled by anxiety and scary thoughts that her new baby will become sick or die.
- One mom realizes that she does not enjoy breastfeeding, and her expectations around this opportunity in motherhood are lost.
- One mom finds that she is unable to enter into her new baby's room without crying, and she suffers great anxiety when she dresses her baby in the clothes that were saved from her first pregnancy.

The experiences go on. Still, similar themes cross over among women and their unique stories. Many of these women are unsure of how to both love their new baby and also grieve the baby they lost. They may feel that they need to choose which baby to be loyal to, and worry that if they become happy and engaged with the baby they brought home, they might, in some way, be forgetting the one who is no longer here.

This confusion and conflict can, in many instances, make it very difficult for these moms to bond and connect with their new babies, no matter how much they have "wanted" them and no matter how much they know they love them despite it all.

While the outside world sees some of these women as first-time mothers, moms in this situation know that they are not. Yet, the story and life of their first child often go unnoticed and are denied by so many. People are unsure of how to talk about infant loss with the women who have this story. Friends, family, and neighbors often become silent rather than reaching out to these moms in an effort to honor the lives of the babies who were lost. The comments that understandably most upset the women whom I work with are those that sound something like this: *"Well, you are young. You can always try for another."* Many of the moms I see have taken this comment as an expectation that another baby is supposed to somehow take the place of the one who was lost. When this is the case, these women may feel neither opportunity, nor the room to be a mother to both.

The way of the mind is complicated, and it fools many of us most of the time. How, on Earth, at a time of such joy can a mom feel so much sorrow? She feels this way because our society does not make much room for grieving and joy together, and we often feel as though we must choose between happiness and sadness—the "either/or" dilemma. Either I am ecstatic to bring a healthy baby home, exude joy, and have "moved on," or I am filled with grief and sorrow and therefore must not love my new baby as I should.

Ugh. What a painful and complicated place to be.

So, my friends, if you are a mom who has experienced miscarriage, stillbirth, or any other loss of an infant or child, please know that the way you feel is normal and valid and real. With support, you can certainly find ways to integrate the baby you lost into your new developing family, and there is, by all means, room to love all of your children. As with most of the work that we do, none of this is easy and it all takes time. There are no "shoulds" around grieving time, and healing is certainly *not* the same as moving on. I encourage self-forgiveness and empathy and understanding and patience with yourself. It is okay to be confused and to miss the dreams and hopes and opportunities that came with the baby who is no longer here. Because I have worked with so many women and have seen shifts and changes occur over and over again, I am quite certain of this: As you make space—perhaps once again—for your conflict and grief and loss, and if you take care of yourself in the process, you will find more room for love and connection and presence with your experience as a mom in *this* moment.

Grieving the Losses and Postpartum Depression Recovery

If only postpartum mood disorders like PPD were as simple as managing symptoms. But of course, the symptoms related to these illnesses—the sadness, tearfulness, the overwhelming intense anxiety, isolation, feelings of hopelessness, irritability, etc.—are only part of the issue, aren't they? Along with these very challenging and often unexpected symptoms comes the double whammy of needing to work through the multitude of losses that accompany perinatal mood and anxiety disorders (PMADs): the loss of self and identity, freedom and independence, energy and sleep, relationships as you know them, expectation and hopes, and, for many, innocence as becoming a parent may be the very first time that a new mom actually feels like a grown-up. For women who have also lost a baby during pregnancy or postpartum or for those women who have experienced deep loss preceding their transition to motherhood, these issues of loss are further complicated. But most women who suffer with a PMAD are dealing with very real losses during this postpartum period. Often, getting through the tangle of symptoms is only a very first step in recovery, and it is the work around grief and loss that requires a mom's most committed attention.

In her book *Therapy and the Postpartum Woman*, Karen Kleiman suggests that women who seek out therapy support during the postpartum period have experienced a "trauma to the soul." Anyone who has struggled through a postpartum mood or anxiety disorder will know, to some degree, what she means by this. Traumas can be defined as "events that cause great distress and disruption," and if becoming a mother does just that and leaves a woman yearning for the parts of herself and her "old life" that are suddenly left behind, her soul can feel as empty as if she has lost something irreplaceable and undeniably valuable to her. I mean, that mom has lost something. Big!

So, how does someone muddle through this very understandable process of grief? While the answer to this varies depending on the particular woman and her own needs with regard to healing, many will go through a series of stages of grief that Elisabeth Kübler-Ross, MD, and David Kessler identified: **denial, anger, bargaining, depression, and acceptance.** Often, these five stages of grief are thought to accompany grief around loss of life. But many, many women who struggle through a PMAD find themselves traveling between these stages as they work to grieve the losses associated with the recent "trauma to their souls."

Let me explain this with some examples.

1. The loss of self and identity:

Denial: I am the same person as I was before I had a baby. I am making too big of a deal about this. I need to just get back to life as normal.

Anger: What is wrong with me?! Where did I go?! Why can't I just manage things as I used to?! I should have never had a baby!

Bargaining: Maybe if I just try a little harder, I will get back to how I was before I had the baby. Maybe if I just pray, then I will find my familiar self.

Depression: I am going to feel like this forever. My life is over, and I will never be happy again.

Acceptance: Maybe parts of me are still here, and maybe I will uncover new pieces of myself that I never knew existed before. Maybe I can decide what kind of mom I want to be without all of the "shoulds" from everyone else. I actually like these parts of myself.

2. The loss of expectation:

Denial: I am happy, I am happy, I am happy, I am happy.

Anger: Why me? Why can't I be content and happy like everyone else? What did I do to deserve this?

Bargaining: Maybe if I just really stick to this attachment parenting practice, I will begin to like it. Maybe if I just breastfeed for one more week, I will feel more like a mom. Maybe if I just do what my own mom says I should do, it will get easier.

Depression: This. Is. Not. Working. I will feel this way forever. I am a total failure.

Acceptance: Okay, so my expectations around new motherhood were unrealistic. Maybe I actually get to have some say in what this looks like for me. Maybe I don't have to follow everyone else's advice, and maybe I can have an experience that works for me, even if it is not what I had expected.

3. The loss of "what was" in a relationship:

Denial: Oh, we are not any different. We are just tired. When we are rested, things will be like they always were.

Anger: He/she doesn't understand me! Why can't he/she just get what I am going through? Why does he/she expect me to want to have sex all the time? His/her life hasn't even changed! This is all his/her fault!

Bargaining: Maybe if I just act as though I am fine, my partner will have confidence in me again. Maybe if I just make myself look prettier, cook more dinners, and pretend to smile more, he/she will like being married/partnered to me again.

Depression: We will never work. Our marriage/partnership will fail. No one will want to be with me because I am sick, sad, unhappy, and incapable.

Acceptance: Okay, other couples go through this. We are not alone. He/she simply does not understand what I am struggling with, and he/she is scared, like me. We are learning new things about each other, and they are not all bad. We can do this. Together.

Ring some bells?

So, this is for all of you who have become moms and, suddenly and unexpectedly, feel that you have lost something. That you are grieving what was. Your work around grieving and then processing these losses is real, and you are not alone. While we know that the five stages of grief are not linear (meaning that the stages can come and go in no particular order), they are all valuable and a part of the process. And resolution comes with allowing yourself to experience each one as it knocks on your door. Even with the gift of a baby can come some very real feelings of loss. And that is okay.

VI. TREATMENT:
Support, Recovery & Finding Joy

Postpartum Depression Recovery: A Therapist's Perspective

Moms know best what they need to get well and to feel like themselves again after postpartum depression. I don't actually mean moms in general, but each one of you. Individually. When it comes to what *you* need to feel well: You. Know. Best.

You know better what you need to feel well than all the postpartum depression books out there (even this one!). You know better than all of your well-intentioned friends and family. You know better than your husband or partner. You even know better than your neighbor or the lady behind you in the checkout line. You. Know. Best.

All of this isn't to say that you should already know what all of your options for recovery are. This is where skilled and trained professionals come in who can guide you on what you might want to consider, what research tells us, and what has worked for others in your shoes. But I'll tell you something, even those of us who are "experts" in the field of perinatal mood and anxiety disorders like postpartum depression don't know ahead of time what the best options might be for each individual mama. You, my friends, are the experts in You.

As I write this, I'm thinking about the moms who sit in my office and "*should*" themselves into a corner. "My own mom says that I should just stay inside and rest, but that makes me feel depressed, and all that I want to do is be outside," says one.

"My husband says I should just quit breastfeeding, but those are actually the only moments that I feel grounded and connected to my baby," says another. "My neighbor says that I should not give my baby formula and that 'breast is best,' but this nursing thing makes me feel trapped and overwhelmed," says the next mama. "Everyone keeps telling me that I should eat three meals each day, but I just can't make that work and find it easier to eat little snacks all day long," says the one after her. "The book I'm reading says that I should wear my baby all the time, but I just want a break!" says the one after that. "And then this other book that I'm reading tells me that I should just let my baby cry, but I get so overwhelmed and anxious," she goes on to say. "I feel like I can't take medication for my depression and anxiety because society says that's a cop-out," so many voices say, "but I am suffering and I've tried everything else already."

Do you see what I mean? Everyone will have advice on what is best for moms in general. Everyone will shout loud and clear about what works for them, and expect that the same thing should be appropriate for others. New advice often contradicts what you have heard only moments before.

When a mom is depressed or anxious, she often feels that she has lost herself, that she no longer knows what is best for her, that she can't make decisions, and that everyone else has the answers before she does. I dare to differ. While I know that it *feels* this way and that symptoms of depression and anxiety can pile up on top of your clearest sense of self and get in the way of your expertise of You, underneath it all you know more than anyone else what will allow you to feel whole again. Many of us are here to help guide you along that path, to work with you to answer your own questions, and to educate you on what we know about treatment options and the pros and cons of each of those. Many of us are here to partner with you as you dig underneath the symptoms to regain that clear sense of yourself. And, at the same time, you are allowed to choose what resonates and what does not; what feels best and what does not.

You get to choose.

What If I Have PPD and Don't Want to Take Meds?

I work with women in my Boulder, Colorado, psychotherapy practice, and most of them are struggling in one way or another with their transition to motherhood. While the range of challenges varies, the desire to feel differently is pretty consistent. Whether a woman is trying to conceive, pregnant, newly postpartum, or more "seasoned" in motherhood, she always sits in my office and says that she wishes she felt better.

"How long will it take?"

"When will I feel better?"

"Will I ever feel like myself again?"

And then, almost always, "Do I have to go on meds?"

Usually, after I learn a bit more about her individual feelings on the issue, my answer to this question is "only if you choose to." While many moderate to severe perinatal mood disorders such as postpartum psychosis and postpartum OCD really do require medication in order to balance out brain chemistry, many perinatal mood and anxiety disorders (PMADs) such as milder forms of postpartum depression and postpartum anxiety can be supported through psychotherapy and other complimentary treatments shown to decrease symptoms.

But it is important that each mom knows the facts. I am a strong believer that each woman knows what is the best course of treatment for herself and her family, but it is important that she understands the specifics of her choices before she makes one. Many women say they don't want to take medication, for example, without knowing that many antidepressants are known to be safe for pregnant and nursing moms.

So, below is some information on the options. While all of these options are known to be effective in treating PPD, it is important to note that usually a combination of treatment modalities is the most comprehensive way to go. Without a doubt, psychotherapy is an important piece of the puzzle, as it offers a safe space to receive validation and support, education, case management, self-care strategy building, and, when necessary, the processing of important family of origin or previous trauma histories that may be contributing to a mom's feelings of being overwhelmed.

Individual Psychotherapy: Weekly therapy with a licensed psychotherapist trained in working with postpartum mood disorders is, as mentioned, an important piece of treatment. This therapist will take a thorough history and help you to identify key pieces of your physical, psychological, and social worlds that may be contributing to your suffering. This therapist will ask you important questions about both how you feel now as well as how you have felt in the past in order to better understand how having a baby or children has affected you. He or she will take a thorough family history that includes both aspects of physical as well as emotional health. He or she will evaluate your basic needs (sleep, nutrition, social support) and help you strategize about ways to fill the gaps, if they exist. This therapist may play an active role in providing other referrals and collaborating with other providers in your community to better support you (such as an OBGYN/midwife, psychiatrist, postpartum doula, acupuncturist, massage therapist or other body workers, nutritionist, pediatrician, parenting coach, or lactation consultant). He or she will help you to set concrete goals toward a greater feeling of health and wellness.

Couples Therapy: Experiencing conflict in a marriage or partnership can be a contributing factor to emotional vulnerability and overwhelm, and having a new baby almost always shakes up feelings of stability. Working with a psychotherapist who is trained in couples work can be an incredibly rewarding piece of the treatment for many women. While it is important to realize that it is totally normal for conflict to arise after having a baby, it is also important to pay attention to this without assuming that things will clear up on their own. A couples' therapist can help to mediate conflict, reset expectations within a relationship, and offer new perspective that can help to get a couple back on track quickly. The strongest marriages are often those that have worked with a therapist during periods of vulnerability. A parenting team is, without doubt, an important piece of family health.

Group Therapy: Mom and baby groups and more structured PPD support groups offer a space for community and support that is invaluable. Usually, these groups will be led by a trained and licensed psychotherapist, other birth or medical professionals, or moms who have recovered from PPD. Connecting with other women at this time can be validating, offer important perspective, and provide community when it might be otherwise lacking. **Psychopharmacology (i.e., antidepressant and anti-anxiety medication):** Misinformation exists about the safety of antidepressant medication during pregnancy and while breastfeeding, and as a result, many women are told that they need to go off their antidepressant medication if they become pregnant. Other breastfeeding moms who suffer from extreme depression and/or anxiety postpartum are told that going on a medication to help with these symptoms is not a possibility. The truth around this is that we know that untreated depression and anxiety can pose more serious risk to a fetus or baby than the potential risks from medication. Babies and children with mothers whose severe depression and anxiety was untreated are at a pretty high risk of developing delays in their emotional, social, and cognitive development. The risks to a baby whose mother is taking medication for her symptoms are low. There are, in fact, many safe and effective medications that moms who are suffering can take when needed. If you choose to take medication, you can usually expect to begin to feel better within two to three weeks, and it is recommended that you remain on your medication for at least six months after you feel better. To learn more about medication while pregnant or breastfeeding, visit the Massachusetts General Hospital's

Center for Women's Health website at womensmentalhealth.org/specialty-clinics/breastfeeding-and-psychiatric-medication/.

Acupuncture: In a study of pregnant women who were diagnosed with major depressive disorder, researchers at Stanford University School of Medicine found that women who received eight weeks of psychotherapy along with acupuncture treatment specific to depression were more likely to see a 50 percent or greater reduction in depressive symptoms than those women who received only psychotherapy or psychotherapy along with generalized acupuncture. This is great news for women who choose not to go the medication route. As with any medical professional you seek, it is important to find an acupuncturist who is familiar with and experienced in the specifics of PPD.

Nutritional Consultation: Pregnancy, childbirth, and nursing are hugely depleting on a mom's nutritional reserves. While a baby will get all that he or she needs from you, it is important that you replenish yourself with important nutrients so your body doesn't become depleted through your generous donations to your baby. We know that nutrient depletion can play a big role in a mom's emotional vulnerability and the development of PPD, so it's crucial to make sure you're giving yourself the important nutritional building blocks for serotonin and other "feel good hormones." A study done at Penn State University and published in *The Journal of Nutrition* found a connection between maternal anemia and the development of PPD, while additional research has found a connection between PPD and lower levels of omega-3 fatty acids. Further, a study published in the *Archives of General Psychiatry* found that PPD may be associated with higher levels of a brain protein called monoamine oxidase A (MAO-A), which removes chemicals that stabilize mood. This study suggests that taking nutrient supplements specific to the proteins lost through MAO-A may help to prevent PPD. Working with a trained professional around some of these issues can lead to better mood and increased ability to sleep for many women.

In addition to the above, other supports known to aid in decreasing symptoms of depression and anxiety include mild to moderate exercise, yoga, and meditation.

A Non-Pharmaceutical Prescription for Symptoms of Postpartum Depression and Anxiety

Although it would be hugely reassuring if we could pinpoint one specific cause of perinatal mood and anxiety disorders like PPD, experts in the field have not yet been able to definitely determine what causes these issues. Actually, what we have found in all of the research and observation is that many factors need to be taken into consideration when we try to assess what it is that is causing a mom to suffer. Here are some of the things we know:

- Major hormone shifts that occur during pregnancy and childbirth likely affect brain chemistry.
- Physiological stressors associated with new parenting (like sleep deprivation and nutrient depletion) affect brain function.
- "Negative thoughts" (including all-or-nothing thinking, should statements, perfectionist thinking, and catastrophic thoughts) impact emotion.
- The major life transition that occurs when becoming a parent requires identity shifting that feels overwhelming.
- Environmental factors surrounding birth (like relationship conflicts, financial struggles, sick newborns, older siblings, traumatic birth, and other major losses and gains) impact emotional stability.
- Lacking or inadequate social networks impact feelings of well-being.

We talk often about treatment and support options for moms who struggle with PMADs, including the often-important role of medication that helps support healthy brain functioning. But now I would like to focus on what I will call a "non-pharmaceutical prescription for mental health." Please understand before reading any further that the discussion below does not suggest that these considerations be used as an alternative to medication; in many cases when symptoms are moderate to severe, medication support is an imperative piece of the treatment picture. However, sometimes we overlook other important factors that impact brain health. We may actually have more control over our brains' physiological response to stress than we think.

Each mom in my office walks away from her first or second session with a non-pharmaceutical prescription. Much research discusses the impact that the following has on brain health and emotional well-being.

1. **Sleep.** It's imperative for brain functioning, no? One study published in the *Archives of Women's Mental Health* suggested that women who got less than four hours of uninterrupted sleep at night were more likely to develop symptoms of PPD than those who achieved this. Without adequate sleep, our

brains cannot function as we need them to, and we are likely to feel less rational and more reactive to stress around us. So, the baseline I give the moms in my office is to strive for at least four hours of uninterrupted sleep (ideally more than that) a night as a part of this prescription.

2. **Nutrition.** Serotonin, the neurotransmitter responsible for emotional wellness, is not free-forming in our bodies, which means that we need to ingest its building blocks in order for it to be produced. The building blocks of serotonin come from amino acids, specifically tryptophan, which can be increased in the brain by eating certain foods and nutrients. This is a much more complicated process than I am able to write about here, but the reality is that eating protein-rich foods that contain tryptophan (meat, poultry, dairy, and nuts) along with carbohydrate-dense foods allows non-serotonin-forming amino acids to be absorbed in the body and tryptophan to be absorbed in the brain, thereby providing the brain with what it needs to produce serotonin. Make sense? Adequate supplies of B6 are also thought to help the process of tryptophan conversion to serotonin. So, eat up.
3. **Water.** Dehydration can cause anxiety as our brains need water to thrive (doesn't everything?). Many, many new moms are dehydrated, especially if they are breastfeeding. Fill that water bottle.
4. **Exercise.** Again, research is overwhelmingly in favor of exercise to both prevent and treat symptoms of depression and anxiety. Of course, during pregnancy and early postpartum, exercise may look more like "movement" than actually running or working out at the gym. But, no doubt, exercising aids in the release of endorphins that play a role in feelings of wellness, reduces the stress hormone cortisol, and assists in important basic need functions such as sleep and appropriate appetite.
5. **Breath.** Sometimes we forget that our brains need oxygen to thrive. When we are feeling anxious, overwhelmed, scared, or distressed, we are usually taking shorter-length chest breaths and are, in doing so, reducing the amount of oxygen to our brains. Deep, long belly breaths (also known as diaphragmatic breathing) can literally change our body's physiological reaction to a stressful situation by encouraging the brain to relax and slow down. Practicing your ability to breathe fully on a daily basis can make this tool more accessible when needed most.
6. **Play.** Yes, play. Research has shown us that play (an activity that is done purely for pleasure, with no focus on a need to accomplish something for someone else) is an anecdote for depression. Thinking outside of the box here can be helpful. Singing in the shower? Dancing in the kitchen? Riding your kid's scooter down the block? Going nuts with the sidewalk chalk? Anything counts.

So, mamas, if you haven't already incorporated them into your lifestyle, you may want to consider which of the above six things are missing for you. Sometimes, women will find that by paying attention to this "prescription," they notice subtle changes in mood that lead to a relief of symptoms of depression and anxiety.

How Does Psychotherapy for Postpartum Depression Work?

I mean how does it *really* work, inside the brain?

It's a very common question.

As many of you can relate, a large percentage of the new moms who come to my therapy practice have never been in therapy before. Although these women may have had symptoms of anxiety or depression in the past, they have been able to manage their symptoms through exercise, managing expectations, ensuring (apparent) control, and other coping behaviors. But now, with a baby in hand, these strategies no longer work, and they find themselves in the last place they expected themselves to be after giving birth: a therapist's office.

Because this setting is so unexpected and new, many of these women enter our work together doubting the process. *Does therapy really work? What is the point of talking about how I am feeling? Is it really going to get me somewhere?*

Psychotherapy treatment for a postpartum illness, at least initially, is often different from therapy for more generalized disorders in that it is very focused on symptom relief. The truth is that many women who come to therapy after having a baby are not seeking long-term psychodynamic support. They are in our offices, rather, because they want—no, they *need*—to feel better. So, our first goal is to work with them to reduce their symptoms. While that is sometimes less simple than it might seem, the first part of PPD treatment is to assess brain chemistry, sleep, nutrition, support, hydration, and exercise so that a mom can do whatever is within her control to help herself to feel better.

Moms who are depressed or anxious also tend to engage in thought patterns that are destructive and ultimately add to their feelings of distress. Because of this, therapy treatment for postpartum depression frequently involves a magnified look at self-talk and the ways in which fortune telling, catastrophic thinking, discounting coping skills, all-or-nothing thinking, overestimating the threat, "what if" statements, and "should" statements (all known clinically as "cognitive distortions") are interfering with a mom's ability to feel good.

Finally, once a mom is feeling well enough to engage in more triggering discussions around her past that may be contributing to her current distress, therapeutic treatment for PPD often looks at beliefs and behaviors that are developed through earlier experiences.

Ahh, this last one: This is where the resistance, hesitation, uncertainty, and often anxiety come in. *Is this talking part really helpful? How much good can talking about what is over and past and done with have in feeling better today?*

So, for this question, let me explain in as basic a way as I can how the brain works.

Our brains are made up of a number of different regions that control logical thinking and rational thought (the prefrontal cortex), emotional processing (the midbrain or limbic system), and the autonomic nervous system or our fight/flight response (the brain stem). Our brains are also divided into two parts: the right hemisphere (responsible for emotion, relational response, and creativity) and the left hemisphere (responsible for abstract and practical thinking).

Experiences that we have, beginning in childhood, help to develop neural pathways, or well-tread patterns, between parts of the brain. Sometimes these neural pathways serve us. For example, if we have been raised by consistent, present, and emotionally available parents, we may learn that others are to be trusted and enter into adult relationships with this assumption. In other words, we develop the instinct to trust.

Sometimes, however, our brains form neural pathways that were once very helpful but that now get in the way of our adult-brained emotional health. This is the case when, for example, a child is raised in an environment in which she is constantly ridiculed, laughed at, and invalidated. This child's brain will, most likely, form neural pathways that lead her to believe as an adult that she should not express herself, that she does not have anything important to say, and that she is not good enough just as she is. For this mom, self-doubt may have become instinctive. At one point she may have been taught this belief by her experiences; it may have once been in her best interest of survival to stay quiet and defer to others. But now? Now that belief does not serve her health and wellness.

So, to frame this very visually, imagine that you are exploring the deep jungle. The grasses are high and the vegetation thick. The path, however, is well-trodden; the grass has been walked on and a clear trail lies ahead. What will you do? You will take this path. It is "easiest" and most traveled, and you know it well. Why on Earth would you try to get to where you are going by bushwhacking through thick and intimidating vegetation?

The answer to *that* question is because, although the path is visible and well-trodden, it no longer takes you to a safe place. It seems easier to take this path, but really where it takes you is to a place that doesn't feel so great.

Yet the rest of the terrain looks impossible to pass through. What you learn in therapy is to form new neural pathways, or new trails, so that instincts and belief systems change for the better. What therapy does is help you to tread a new path in the vegetation, often step by step, little by little, until a new trail is formed—one that takes you to someplace that feels good. And what happens over time to that old path? As it is walked on less and less, the grasses return to where they once were and, over time, that trail no longer exists.

A well-trained psychotherapist helps with this process by working with you to explore these old patterns. Talking about this stuff allows you to gain the information you need to understand why you think and behave the way you do today. And once you understand the implications of early experiences, you are armed with the awareness—and hopefully the tools—to trail blaze someplace new.

This is not always easy, of course. But physical strength (obtained through basic needs), unconditional support and encouragement (from your therapist, your spouse, or others close to you), and the prospect of a happier way of being make this all very, very possible.

Through therapy, you literally change the landscape and structure of your brain. So, yes, according to brain science, therapy does work.

Eight Types of Psychotherapy for Postpartum Depression Treatment

You've probably heard it before: One of the best ways to treat a postpartum mood and anxiety disorder like postpartum depression is through therapy. "Find a therapist" is probably the first suggestion you will hear from people who specialize in these challenges. Symptoms of depression, anxiety, post-traumatic stress, OCD, and adjustment can be understood, worked through, and alleviated through psychotherapy, but what this treatment looks like can vary tremendously.

So, what is psychotherapy, exactly? While a Licensed Clinical Social Worker (LCSW), Licensed Professional Counselor (LPC), Marriage and Family Therapist (MFT), and Psychologist (PsyD or PhD) can all provide psychotherapy support, what this support looks like may be different depending on that particular therapist's approach to treatment. "I am seeing a therapist" can mean something very different for each person.

To provide some clarity around this, let's discuss the different types of therapy that are most utilized in the treatment of a postpartum mood and anxiety disorder like postpartum depression.

Interpersonal Psychotherapy (IPT)

Interpersonal Psychotherapy is currently thought to be one of the most effective therapy models for treating PPD. IPT is a time-limited form of therapy (12 to 16 weeks), and the main goal is symptom relief. An IPT therapist tends to be direct and active in the treatment, and he or she will help to make insights regarding the sources of a new mom's distress. IPT is based on the premise that postpartum distress is rooted in four "problem areas":

- Grief: Acknowledging the losses that occur to sense of self, changes in relationships, or more specific loss.
- Role Transitions: Life stage transitions and social transitions including loss of independence and changing social networks.
- Interpersonal Disputes: Ones that frequently occur after the birth of a child, including unmet expectations and intimacy struggles within partnerships.
- Interpersonal Deficits: Looking at struggles with attachment in other relationships that may be causing distress.

A big part of IPT is the teaching of communication skills that assist in building relationships, stronger social support, and increased confidence. IPT is manual-based and follows a specific course of treatment.

Cognitive Behavioral Therapy (CBT)

CBT is best known for its efficacy in treating anxiety disorders such as OCD. CBT works with the understanding that the way we think affects the way that we feel, and so treatment is focused on helping mom have control over her thoughts so that she feels more able to change them. A CBT therapist will work with a mom to identify and acknowledge her automatic thoughts, evaluate these thoughts, and become aware of when these thoughts are not helpful; explore and change underlying beliefs; differentiate between realistic and false threats; and develop new and more helpful perspectives. CBT helps a mom to develop coping strategies so she feels better equipped to manage distress. CBT uses tools such as homework, relaxation, exposure therapy, thought stopping, mental imagery, and tools for changing catastrophic thoughts and irrational thinking. Mindfulness-Based Cognitive Therapy (MBCT) is a form of CBT that also incorporates mindfulness meditation.

Dialectical Behavioral Therapy (DBT)

DBT began as a treatment for borderline personality disorder but is now known to be effective in many instances where distress is prominent. Like CBT, DBT uses practice and homework as a part of its process. DBT teaches skills in the following categories: mindfulness, distress tolerance, emotional regulation, and interpersonal effectiveness. DBT focuses on the role of feelings and emotion in distress (as opposed to the thoughts that CBT focuses on). DBT is often supported through both group and individual therapy and follows a specific guideline for teaching skills to reduce symptoms related to distress.

Psychodynamic Psychotherapy

Psychodynamic Psychotherapy is one of the earliest types of psychotherapy and focuses on unconscious and past experiences in understanding current behavior. Psychodynamic psychotherapists believe that our earliest childhood experiences have a direct impact on our present distress, and that when moms can identify and accept these experiences as playing a role, they are able to begin the process of healing and becoming less entangled in the past. This type of therapy looks into early experiences that play a role in forming beliefs about ourselves as adults, and identifies those beliefs that are no longer helpful. When working with a psychodynamic psychotherapist, a mom will be encouraged to talk about her relationships with her parents and other significant people to uncover the unconscious content of a mom's way of thinking, being, and relating to others. This process reduces tension and distress. A psychodynamic approach to treatment is thought to be important because change requires awareness and understanding to occur. Often in this type of therapy, the "aha" moments allow for self-validation, empathy, and, ideally, freedom from self-judgment.

Eye Movement Desensitization and Reprocessing (EMDR)

EMDR is currently thought to be one of the most effective types of therapy when working through a traumatic experience and is being used more in the treatment of postpartum PTSD. This specialized type of therapy requires specific training and credentialing. EMDR uses elements of both CBT and Psychodynamic Psychotherapy along with specific techniques that are used to reduce the sensory impact of traumatic memories. Because traumatic memories are often stored in either the right (feeling-based and emotional) or left (logical and intellectual) side of the brain, EMDR uses a bilateral stimulation of the brain (through eye movements, bilateral sound, or bilateral tactile stimulation) combined with beliefs, visualization, and attention to body awareness to reprocess memories more effectively. A significant piece of EMDR involves helping mom to access thoughts and feelings that are positive, grounding, and healing.

Solution-Focused Brief Psychotherapy

Solution-Focused Brief Psychotherapy focuses on a specific issue and works toward positive change. Unlike other therapies that identify early experiences as playing a role in current distress, solution-focused therapy stays away from past problems and instead highlights a mom's strengths and skills. Much of this type of therapy is about setting goals and is solution-based rather than problem-solving. This very short-term therapy often requires several sessions to be beneficial; however, many other types of clinicians may feel that this type of therapy does not address the root cause of problems effectively enough to create lasting change.

Group Therapy

Group Therapy uses the role of community in support. A true group therapy session is facilitated by one or more trained psychotherapists and uses the dynamics that occur between members of the group to help identify problem areas and interpersonal distress. A postpartum depression support group often combines psycho-education (teaching about maternal mental illnesses, causes, treatment options, life strategies for wellness, typical new mom stresses, etc.) with the important role of validation from others in the group. The goal of a PPD support group is to help build community, to give space for a mom to be heard by others and learn that she is not alone in her struggles, and to talk about and share ideas regarding stress management, coping, and early mothering.

Couples Therapy

Couples Therapy provides a space for partners to be heard during a time of crisis. In a couples therapy setting, recurrent negative patterns within the relationship will be addressed, and couples will learn communication and listening strategies necessary in working through these challenges. Often in postpartum work, couples therapy will address issues related to PMADs, changing dynamics in a relationship, intimacy challenges, individual needs that may be interfering with connection, and individual needs that are necessary in maintaining the health of a couple's relationship.

When interviewing new therapists, it is absolutely appropriate to ask each therapist what type of therapy he or she practices. However, in most cases you will find that therapists use pieces of many different types of therapy in their work. A therapist who has a specific training and therapeutic background may allow for other types of therapy in his or her work when working with a mom struggling with a PMAD. Specialists in the treatment of PMADs will be driven by what is known about important aspects in PMAD treatment (biological causes, symptom reduction, life change management, expectation, infant-attachment support, etc.) and will either incorporate therapeutic approach into this work or wait to begin that phase of treatment until a mom's initial distress is managed.

Ten Things to Know about Psychotherapy Treatment for PPD

Every time a mom in distress calls me to schedule a new therapy appointment, I am reminded of the courage this takes. Society just doesn't set us up for the reality of needing this type of support after having a baby. Women are led to envision romantic moments around breastfeeding, moments cradling a swaddled baby who sleeps peacefully with a light smile on her lips, loving and contented embraces with partners, and sweet jaunts through the park with a baby carriage in which a baby lies peacefully.

Certainly, these moments may happen, but more times than not, new parents find themselves in the midst of moments that feel less ideal than these. Very few women spend time envisioning themselves nestled into a therapist's couch when they look forward to the first weeks and months of being a mother.

However, psychotherapy is known to be one of the most important types of treatment for women with moderate to severe symptoms of depression and anxiety during pregnancy or postpartum.

So recalling all of these brave calls to my office, I share this list of 10 things to keep in mind when you are considering reaching out to a trained psychotherapist for support.

Sometimes making the first call is the hardest part. Women tell me all the time that they have been holding onto my card for months. Acknowledging that you cannot heal on your own, picking up the phone to ask for help, and disclosing your most intimate information for the first time to someone you don't know can be excruciatingly difficult. But once you do take this step, you may find that you begin to feel better immediately.

Therapists who are appropriately trained in treating postpartum mood and anxiety disorders like PPD won't judge you. Chances are, no matter how awful you believe that your symptoms, thoughts, or behaviors sound, a skilled therapist will have heard it already. Many women will resist psychotherapy for fear that their therapist will think awful things about them, and this is unfortunate. Give your therapist a chance to hear you out and understand.

Yes, therapy is hard work, and it doesn't always feel good. One of the important pieces of healing from PPD involves talking openly about how you feel, what you are thinking, and parts of your environment that might be contributing to your distress. And, often, it feels easiest (and less painful) to keep these things stored inside where nobody can touch them. However, the way past this kind of distress is through it, and an appropriately trained therapist will support you in a way that feels gradual and safe.

I often relate psychotherapy to physical therapy that is used to treat a physical injury, like a knee injury. In order to heal a knee injury, you may need to go into a physical therapist's office and move your knee in ways that feel painful in the moment. Your knee may feel additionally sore for a time. However, with work and treatment, your knee begins to strengthen and heal. Psychotherapy and the brain work the same way.

The time and resources that you give to your individual therapy will serve your whole family. Often, women talk about how "selfish" it feels to be spending money or time away from their baby in order to be at a therapy session. Yet this does not take into account the impact that your own healing will have on those around you. Through your own work at healing, your relationships with your partner (or family and friends) and your attachment with your baby will strengthen. Sometimes it takes the realization that "I am going to therapy *for* my baby and family" to actually motivate women to pick up the phone.

If you don't gel with your therapist, it is entirely appropriate to seek out someone else whom you feel more comfortable with. For most therapists, what matters is that you get the kind of support you need to heal, not that it must be a specific one of us who supports you in this healing. It can be hard to have this conversation with a new therapist, but most of us will be more than willing to help you connect with someone different if the chemistry doesn't feel like a fit for you. With this said, it is also important to talk through your concerns with a new therapist before deciding that he or she won't be able to support you. You may find a misunderstanding somewhere (by you or your therapist) that can be worked out easily.

Often, your therapist may ask you to sign something that gives him or her permission to talk with other important people in your life (OBs, MDs, midwives, pediatricians, doulas, lactation consultants, psychiatrists, acupuncturists, other medical providers, and/or family). If this request is made, please understand that it is to best serve you in your treatment—to enable the therapist to create a comprehensive team of support people so that things don't fall between the cracks. Sometimes this release of information can feel scary, but you will find that enabling the therapist to talk openly with select others about your care enhances the support you will receive.

If medication is a part of your treatment plan, please understand the value of psychotherapy support along with this. Sometimes a medication to treat postpartum depression or anxiety will work so well to decrease or eliminate symptoms that women will feel that therapy is no longer needed. While brain chemistry imbalance is often a large "cause" of postpartum distress, not addressing the other physical, psychological, and/or social contributions to a mom's challenges is, in my opinion, a missed opportunity. Medication is often an important part of symptom relief, but a lifelong change in mental health will almost always involve aspects that go beyond the medication you are taking.

What you learn in your therapy treatment about managing anxiety and depression will be a gift. I know tit probably doesn't feel like that now, but you will likely walk away from your therapy with tools that you can pass down to your kiddos that will help them to manage distress in their own lives. Life can be stressful, and many of us don't learn the skills to manage distress until we are well into adulthood. Through you, your children can learn some of those skills early, and this will serve them immensely throughout their lifetimes.

Your therapy support will probably include a combination of education around perinatal mood and anxiety disorders; talking through how you feel; coming up with a plan that involves physical, social, and emotional strategies for health; and valuable support while you negotiate the journey toward wellness. And while you understandably would like to feel better immediately, this takes time.

You will feel better with support. When women reach out to an appropriately trained mental health provider, follow treatment recommendations, and stick with the treatment, they get well. All the time.

Ten Things a Mom Learned in Therapy That Led Her to Emotional Health

I love the work that I do... truly! Recently, a woman with whom I work in my Boulder psychotherapy practice reminded me of this once again. What this phenomenal woman reminded me of is this: Emotional pain is excruciating, but even depression that keeps someone in a place of deep despair for much of a lifetime can be shifted. Not easily, of course, but with hard work, commitment, insight, and hope, heaviness can be lifted, and emotional health recovered.

With her permission, I'd like to share her list with you of the 10 things she has realized are important for her to feel well. Ten things she says that she learned in my office, but 10 things that, truthfully, she has discovered on her own.

1. Pay attention to physical health and symptom reduction. Like so many others, Lisa (not her real name) spent years in doctors' offices seeking help for what she believed was physical illness. Emotional pain can be stored in the body and identified initially as physical ailments that seem ongoing. When insomnia, body pain, and other physical distractions seem unexplainable and chronic, depression and/or anxiety may be the cause. Lisa spent much of her life seeking help for these issues but now realizes that the cause of many of them was her emotional stress and depression. What she has found is that when she takes care of herself physically (through sleep, nutrition, exercise, and breath), she feels better emotionally. As she recovers from her depression, she feels less physical pain and discomfort.

2. Acknowledge, defend, and obtain wants and needs. Lisa is not unlike so many others who have been motivated by the *shoulds* in life. Lisa has been so accustomed to this that it took some time for her to recognize what her own *wants* and *needs* are outside of the *shoulds* placed on her by others. When Lisa was able to listen carefully to her own internally driven wants and needs, she found that she not only accessed important instincts, but she also was more likely to achieve her goals. She has found that she needs to speak up for herself in this area, and she has learned to be her own advocate regardless of the expectations of others.

3. Self-monitor and self-soothe. Lisa learned the importance of listening for changes in the way she feels. What she found is that when she can notice shifts in body tension, her thought processes, and her reactions to things, she is able to catch her rising stress early enough to stop it in its tracks. Lisa has found deep breathing to be an especially helpful tool, along with other coping strategies for emotional health such as taking a break, exercise, and getting outdoors.

4. Accept emotional turbulence and understand that suffering is temporary. As a child, Lisa was not allowed to feel anything other than happiness. Struggle (especially fear, sadness, and anger) was not welcome in her household. Because of this,

Lisa had learned to dread the negative emotions that are experienced in life. Each time that she experienced even "normal" amounts of distress, she was catapulted into a deep, dark hole that she felt she could not get out of. Through our work together, Lisa learned that emotional turbulence is a normal part of being human, and that if she can let go of the need to change or deny it, her suffering is temporary. This awareness has lifted the additional layer of stress and self-judgment she often felt whenever she experienced anything other than happiness. This has made the suffering she does experience from time to time more tolerable.

5. Have self-compassion and be nonjudgmental. Along with the above, Lisa has learned to understand the devastating impact that self-judgment has had on her well-being. As she learned to understand why she has felt the way she has with compassion and empathy for herself, her confidence and acceptance of herself has grown immensely.

6. Take pride and find value in one's actions and life. When she first came into my office, Lisa described who she was and her actions in life as less than adequate. She was quick to criticize herself and her role in her life and felt the ongoing effects of this on her mood. Over time, however, Lisa has realized much goodness in who she is and what she does, and this awareness has brought about a level of joy that she had not yet discovered. She often asks herself, "How do I perceive what I am doing?" When she notices that she is holding a view that is critical, she also becomes aware that this is probably not accurate. By learning to shift her perspectives, she has also learned to value herself.

7. Be your own mother. I think many of you can relate. Lisa did a wonderful job working to be a "good mother" to her daughter, but she missed the boat on taking care of herself. Throughout our work together, Lisa realized more and more that much of her struggle was because she was not getting what she needed to be well, and that she would never treat her daughter the way she was treating herself. A focus on her own basic needs as well as how she is speaking to herself has helped her to thrive.

8. Maintain social contact when down. When I first met Lisa, she described herself as "socially awkward" and as someone who preferred to be alone. But what we realized together was that being alone was actually something that had occurred as an (unhealthy) coping response to her depression. When Lisa felt depressed, she pulled away from others, and yet the isolation she felt as a result of this only increased her feelings of despair. One of the first things she now does when she's feeling down is to reach out to someone whom she trusts for company and support for her emotional health, even when her instinct is to pull away.

9. Be curious. When we first met, Lisa was quick to label herself and her feelings, but she has learned over time to be curious rather than critical. Instead of telling herself that something she feels or a choice she makes is "bad," she instead asks herself "why" she feels the way she feels or made the choice she did. By asking questions, she has found that opportunities for understanding and growth are limitless. She has found great meaning and insight in who she is through this curiosity.

10. Balance play, rest, work, and reflection. Lisa has been an "all-or-nothing" thinker for much of her life. She has found that she tends toward either all work, all play, or all rest (in her most depressed times this resulted in her spending all day in bed), and that she had never even considered the value of reflection that wasn't all self-critical. In our initial work together, she often tried to define herself by one of the above ways of being (I am a "doer," I am a "worker," or I am "lazy"). What she found is that she needs all the above to thrive, and that when she focuses on only one way of being, she misses out on the rest. "Balance" to Lisa has not meant equal parts throughout a day as much as it's meant that she allows space for each. When she feels that she is leaning too far in one direction, she pauses and asks herself what she needs now to even out the imbalances.

So many women who seek support and treatment for their depression and anxiety uncover much of what Lisa has, but something remarkable existed in how she put it all together this way. In doing so, Lisa created a recipe for herself that she can now follow when she needs her own guidance. Doing so is not always easy for her; when someone has a long history of mental illness like depression, there is no quick fix toward wellness. **Being well is a practice that demands attention and focus.** But she is on her way. I am moved by her clarity and determination. And her willingness to share what she has learned with others.

Three cheers!

Five Common Concerns about Therapy for Postpartum Depression

Ask any clinician who treats postpartum depression and related illnesses, and they'll tell you that many times when a mom who is struggling and in desperate need of support reaches out for an initial therapy session, she does not return. And while those of us who get the cancellation call or who wait in our offices at the time of her appointment until we register that she is not coming feel worried or disappointed that we will not see her again, we also get it. This postpartum depression treatment stuff is hard. And it can be scary. And it can feel like another mountain to climb when a mom is already worn out from the first several mountains she has encountered since giving birth to her baby.

Sometimes it may be that we simply weren't the best fit for this particular mom who finally reached out for help with PPD and is now disheartened by the idea that no one can help her.

A mom cancels after a first session and we understand why. Nonetheless, it still concerns us, because while some of these moms may reach out again or seek out someone better fitted to their personalities or needs, many will never attempt to get support after that first appointment. These moms will walk away from that first session with a variety of concerns about therapy for postpartum depression. Among them are these five thoughts:

1. "No way am I doing *that* again. If I go back and see her, she will make me take medication, and I'm not doing that."
2. "I knew I shouldn't have tried therapy. I knew he would just ask me about my own parents, and I am so done talking about them."
3. "When I told her that I was thinking about wanting to hurt myself, the therapist said I needed to let my husband/partner know how much I am struggling. I knew that I couldn't trust her to keep my secrets."
4. "He suggested that I need more time for myself? What does he know?! I don't have more time for myself. Clearly, he does not understand..."
5. "It's just too expensive. I can't afford her fee every week, so I will never be able to get support."

I, like many others, understand these concerns, but I am also concerned for those moms who, because of the frustrations they walk away with, never receive adequate treatment and care. What we know without a doubt is that moms who reach out for support from an appropriately trained expert in perinatal mental health and who follow treatment recommendations get well.

So, what to do about these very valid concerns if you find yourself cancelling after a first session? Go back, at least one more time, and talk about them. As hard as this might be. You see, the truth is that the first session is not necessarily an adequate representation of the work because connections, trust, and assessments can take time.

If you don't agree with your therapist's suggestion to take medication, ask her why she feels that medication is important for you and help her to understand what concerns you about this option. If you are frustrated by his questions about your own family, let him know that so he can identify the reasons why this piece of history may be important in understanding your current struggles as a mom. If you are angry that she isn't willing to keep your suicidal thoughts a secret, tell her this and make space for a conversation regarding why this type of secret is harmful to you. If you feel misunderstood, do your best to be open about who you are and what you are struggling with. If you still feel misunderstood, ask for another referral from that therapist or someone else. Many of us care more that you get the support you need than that you are seeing us for this support. If you cannot afford her fee, ask her about the option of a sliding scale; most of us will have a number of these spots in our practice if we do not accept insurance as direct payment.

You have been through so much already. Postpartum depression is a lonely and often very long battle when you are in it alone. Let us help you get to the support that will lead you toward wellness again.

Six Things You Should Know about Antidepressants and Pregnancy

Those of us who specialize in perinatal mental health wish more than anything that we had more certainty for you—that we had one right answer for everyone so that we could take the burden away from you of having to figure it all out. We know that when you are tired and anxious and overwhelmed and unsure, nothing is more difficult than having to make a decision when the information is complicated and so much unknown exists in the midst of it all. Truthfully, it's not okay that we don't know more, and we need to keep on doing the research necessary to continue to build toward more clarity.

So, what I want to say to you is this: If you are frustrated, we get it. If you are confused, it makes sense. If you are angry, you get to be angry. And if you have questions, ask them.

When you reach out for help from a trained professional, you have a right to know their expertise, their commitment to best practice and professional development, and their loyalty toward helping *you* decide what the best course of action is for your particular situation. Not every mom with postpartum or antenatal depression or anxiety will end up including medication in her treatment plan, but many will. Those of us rooting for you and your babies understand the trust you put in us to help you decide what is the safest and most appropriate way to help your family thrive.

There is a lot of misinformation out there about the risks of taking antidepressants during pregnancy or while breastfeeding. I'd like to address this misinformation with six important facts:

It is not possible or appropriate to make one blanket statement regarding the use of antidepressant medication, such as selective serotonin reuptake inhibitors (SSRIs), during pregnancy (or breastfeeding). These decisions need to be made on a case-by-case basis and must take into account each mom's unique symptoms and family picture.

While some research suggests that SSRIs may not be safe to take during pregnancy, more research suggests that they are. And, when we look closely at this research, the statements made to suggest that SSRIs are dangerous to a fetus are selective and do not account for the whole picture. Another way of saying this is that many of these studies you sometimes see covered by the media are not "clinically sound."

Untreated and under-treated perinatal mood and anxiety disorders can have significant negative effects on a developing baby's social, emotional, and cognitive development. This, by the way, is rarely, if ever, debated.

Sometimes lifestyle changes like increased sleep and nutrition or non-pharmaceutical treatments like acupuncture and light therapy help a mom recover from her symptoms, but sometimes they do not and a more involved treatment like psychotherapy or the use of an SSRI is required for a mom to be well.

Taking an SSRI medication during pregnancy under the guidance of an appropriately trained clinician is not irresponsible.

"Gray area" exists when it comes to the use of SSRI medication during pregnancy and breastfeeding. Many of us are uncomfortable with the "grays" and want instead a more black-and-white, clear answer to these things. While this gray area can be confusing, it does not need to be scary. Instead, we can try to think of the gray as a place for options.

So, moms: On behalf of all of the appropriately trained perinatal mental health specialists out there, I know that these decisions are hard for you and that the choice of whether or not to take medication while you are pregnant or lactating is rarely simple. I believe that you want what is best for your baby (and so do I!), and I'm confident that the choices you make that lead you to wellness will undoubtedly benefit your kiddos in the long run.

Trained perinatal mental health specialists will continue to research the role of pharmaceutical medication in the treatment of perinatal mood and anxiety disorders and will advise you on best practice and sound clinical knowledge. We will not mislead you. We will let you know what we don't know, but we will also let you in on what we do, and we will do this with educated knowledge and research-based understanding.

And, we know that this does not feel easy, although we wish that it were. But you have our promise to continue to learn and push and stand by your side as you do what is required to be your best self. For you and for your baby.

Your Questions Answered about Medication for Postpartum Depression

The absolute last thing you desired or even considered upon having a baby is the need to show up in a psychotherapist's office to talk about postpartum depression. Dreaming about life with a baby usually involves thoughts of long and warm cuddles, peaceful walks with baby carriers, and everlasting happiness and soft, adorable kisses. So, when the realization comes that you may be actually spending week after week on a therapist's couch working through unexpected emotional turbulence rather than on your own with a peaceful baby in your arms, you may feel deep and unrelenting disappointment. And frustration. And a (very valid) "why me??!"

And then? A medication evaluation and possible antidepressant on top of it all? Most new moms certainly were not expecting that. Almost every mom who walks into my office for a first visit says something like, *"I am really, truly suffering. I cannot bear to feel like this anymore. But I am NOT taking an antidepressant!"*

Now, let me disclose here that I live and work in a community where "natural living" is idealized and many women feel an intense pressure to avoid medication whenever possible. But I think it's probably pretty fair to suggest that most new moms are somewhat apprehensive to include medication in their treatment plan, at least initially. When this is the case, I've noticed that the uncertainty usually surrounds several questions:

1. What will it do to my baby if I am breastfeeding?
2. Will it make me happy all the time? Or numb?
3. What are the side effects?
4. Will I have to be on medication forever?
5. Can't I just get through all of this pain and suffering without medication?
6. Isn't taking medication a weakness? It means that I can't do this!

Let's take a closer look at each of these, and I'll try to ease some of this uncertainty.

Most studies have shown that the risk of certain SSRI medications on breastfed babies is extremely low. But we do know that the developmental risks for babies of depressed or anxious moms are high. Because of this, experts who treat postpartum depression and anxiety will say that the risk of untreated depression/anxiety outweighs the potential risk of these medications in breast milk. Like many others in my field, I feel strongly that the absolute best gift we can give our children is our own health and happiness. So, by taking these medications, if you need them, you will most likely be able to be present, be more content, have more energy, and attach and bond to your baby in ways that are undeniably healthy for him or her. Moms may choose to stop breastfeeding when taking their medications, but they don't necessarily need to do so. What will it do to your baby? It will give him his mother back.

Antidepressant medication will not make you happy all the time. It will not take away the fact that caring for a baby is exhausting and at times overwhelming. It will not make you love changing diapers at 3:00 a.m., and it will not ensure that you are a mom who runs cheerfully barefoot with your baby in the freezing rain singing at the top of your lungs (well, maybe). What it will likely do is make it easier for you to sleep at night because your rambling brain will quiet down and stop its noise. What it will do is decrease many of your postpartum depression symptoms so that you feel more motivated, interested, and engaged in things that do make you happy. Medication does not change who you are. It takes away the noise and the pain and the distraction so you can be more of who you are.

The side effects vary from person to person, and if you are struggling with side effects that are intolerable to you, you will probably need to switch to a different medication. The most common side effect that I have seen in my office is a lowered libido, but many women who are depressed or anxious don't really feel like having sex anyway. Sometimes when starting with a new SSRI, some women feel slightly agitated for a few days, but this should be tolerable and the heightened agitation should go away in several days. It is always important to give your doctor a full medical history as women who have a history of bipolar disorder are better served by a mood stabilizer than an antidepressant such as an SSRI (which can often initiate a manic period).

Most people who go on an antidepressant during pregnancy or postpartum do not need to be on that medication forever. Clinically it is important to stay on your medication for at least six months to a year after you begin to feel better, and women who go off sooner than that are much more likely to relapse. Once the brain is functioning more efficiently, it needs time to get used to functioning in this capacity; and you need time to gather all of the stress reduction, mindfulness, and/or cognitive behavioral skills needed to maintain your well-being if and when you decide to go off the medication.

The question of whether you should be able to do this on your own? I get this question all the time. The answer is: not likely if you are suffering from moderate or severe symptoms of depression or anxiety. I have mom after mom in my office who knows exactly what she needs to feel better (be it yoga or exercise or sleep or community), but no matter how hard she tries, she can't make these things happen or she is doing them but they aren't having the desired effect. With each attempt she becomes more depleted, frustrated, and insecure. The thing is that if your brain chemistry is off, no yoga, hike, lunch with a friend, or restless nap is going to make you feel better for very long. When moms in my office who really do need medication in their recovery finally do decide to go that route, they find that they are finally motivated to get to yoga, have the energy for a hike, sleep better, and can think more clearly through the logistics needed for self-care.

From where I sit—and, yes, these things are always much easier said than done—making the decision to take medication if needed is an undeniable strength. It is brave and in service of both self and others. Strength comes from conquering fear and uncertainty, does it not?

I am by no means a "pill pusher," and, in most cases, unless a mom is in real crisis, I believe fully that each mom should be able to make her own choices around her treatment. But what I do want to do is to make sure that each woman who walks into my office is informed, and that those who are quick to deny medication understand why they are making that choice and aren't selling themselves short because of (understandable and hugely challenging) stigma, judgment, and ignorance. Sometimes women suffer for much longer than they need to. More times than not I have heard women say, "If only I had been willing to do this sooner...."

I AM OK

Consider for a moment that the opposite of fear might be confidence. Not safety, but confidence.

Most of us, when we are feeling fear, are in a place where we don't believe that we are okay. We have a sense that we will not survive something that we are faced with. We feel fear in a challenging situation like the loss of a job or a divorce or social pressure or an argument with someone. We feel fear in moments when we don't understand, don't know the answer to something, or are incompetent or ineffective. We fear the discomfort that we feel when we are faced with grief or worry or anger. **If we really pause and take a deep look, we fear annihilation. We fear death. We simply do not believe that we are okay. We lack confidence that we will be able to tolerate the emotional and physical pain that we are experiencing.**

Fear occurs when we lack the confidence that we are okay.

If our definition of "okay" is happy and calm and grounded and together, then, perhaps, we are right.

But what if *being okay* means that we, really, *are* okay even when we are feeling grief or anger or worry or uncertainty? What if we really believed that we could survive the intense discomfort that comes with all of the things listed above? What if we really, truly believed that we were okay even when things were totally awful? **What if way deep down inside we learned to trust our ability to tolerate ourselves and the world around us when shit totally hit the fan?**

In moments of distress, the mantra running through our minds is almost always *"I am not okay."* This takes its toll.

Forgive me for getting spiritual or esoteric here. But you always have been okay. You actually have made it through. Even when things have been horrific and you have felt deep pain, you have survived. *You are okay.*

We can all change our thought patterns to acknowledge this truth. Here is how:

1. Get curious about your definition of *"okay"* Is there room for you to believe that even when you feel deep discomfort, you can survive the moment and get through to the other side?

2. Watch your thoughts in times of distress. Do they lean toward catastrophe and annihilation?

3. Practice a different mantra as often as you can. **I. Am. OK.** Think these words while you are walking. While you are doing the dishes. While you are waiting in line. While you breathe in and while you breathe out.

I. Am. OK.

Too much? Then try this: *What if I am actually okay?*

I am okay *when I go into childbirth and am scared.* ***I am okay*** *when my baby is crying and I don't know why.* ***I am okay*** *when I have to go into an uncomfortable conversation with my partner.* ***I am okay*** *when my child is yelling at me.* ***I am okay*** *when I have to make a parenting decision and I have no idea what to do.* ***I am okay*** *when I am scared or when I am sick or when I am awaiting life-changing news.* ***In this moment, I am okay.***

For those of us who have sustained deep hurt and trauma, this is not easy. Most things aren't. But if you are living in a state of fear and anxiety or deep sadness and depression, I suggest you give it a try. Start with just one week.

I AM OK!!

SELF-CARE AND PRIORITIES

If moms who walk into my office walk out believing one thing, I hope it is that self-care is not gluttonous. That it is not selfish to want time away from their babies. That it is not self-indulgent to get a haircut, or go out to a movie, or take a hot bath, or go see a friend, or, God forbid, get a massage. Self-care is far from selfish. If moms who leave my office do so understanding that taking care of themselves is not just for themselves but also for their babies, then I have succeeded in something.

I had a mom in my practice once tell me that coming to therapy was the first *"self-indulgent thing"* she had done since her son was born six weeks ago. It is amazing to me that, as women and mothers in this society, our own needs for comfort, health, and sanity seem to go flying out the window once our children are born. We go way down on the priority list almost instantly. We are somehow led to believe that we should not matter anymore and that the only way to be a "good mother" is to be selfless and always put our baby's needs first.

Have you ever heard the flight attendant say, oh so casually, to put your mask on first before attempting to help others?

But this does not happen for many new moms. It seems all too common for women to forget to eat nutritious meals, to forgo sleep because they are expected to, to deny themselves the "luxury" of exercise or haircuts or soothing comforts or even therapy. Yet we know that with more sleep, time away, a new haircut, a hearty meal, and some exercise we have more to give to those little beings who rely on us for their every need. When we are tired and depleted and lonely, we are less able to be present with those who need us most.

Depression and anxiety are certainly not a reflection of a mom's desire to parent or the love she has for her baby. But they can, and often do, interfere with her ability to be present and to enjoy the early weeks and months with her baby. One of the many things that can cause someone to feel unsteady emotionally is a void in the things that help her to feel whole: sleep, nutrition, community, exercise, a place to feel validated, a hot shower, space…

So, moms: Put yourself back at the top of that priority list. That simple act is an irreplaceable gift for your baby.

Ten Tips for Dealing with Stress for Moms Who've Had PPD

"But I don't have PPD anymore! I am not supposed to feel depressed or anxious! I should know better than to wake up and feel like I don't want to face the day! What is wrong with me? Does this mean I'm back to where I started?"

Sound familiar?

We are all likely to go through a period of stress at some time or another, and for moms who have struggled through a postpartum mood or anxiety disorder like PPD, these periods can feel downright terrifying (and often way too familiar). Yet they are unavoidable if a mom is in any way human (I know, what a bummer), so understanding what stress-related depression is about and how to take care of yourself in the midst of it is important.

What do we mean by *stress-related depression*? Really, all that this describes is an episode of depression (or anxiety) that is triggered by a stressful event or periods of prolonged stress. In clinical terms we call this *psychosocial stress,* which means that it's caused by disruptions in someone's environment. A mom who is typically healthy can go through something that feels stressful—anything from a new job, an exciting move, a vacation, or building and renovating a house, to illness, financial loss, relationship conflict, or loss of a loved one—and suddenly feel as though she has lost all semblance of mental health and clarity. She can feel as though she is suddenly incapable. Behind. Incompetent. Unable.

Here's the thing, though: Stress itself is neither bad nor abnormal and is, in fact, an entirely acceptable and normal psychological and physiological response to both positive and negative situations in one's life. What matters in mental health is not that you avoid stress, but that you know how to deal with it so the impact of stress doesn't linger. Prolonged stress can lead to increased cortisol and decreased serotonin and dopamine (neurotransmitters responsible for emotional wellness) if it isn't managed well. Without these neurotransmitters and adequate brain functioning, we simply become less resilient to the stress we are facing, and we become symptomatic (tearful, anxious, overwhelmed, fatigued, hopeless, apathetic). This is often what occurs when we aren't mindful about taking care of ourselves *while* we are feeling stressed.

While stress-related depression is not necessarily a relapse of postpartum depression, we do know that moms who struggle with PPD are usually those whose brains are genetically more vulnerable to imbalances in brain chemistry. Moms who struggle and recover from PPD may need to be mindful of self-care and emotional wellness throughout their lifetimes. This does not mean that they are certain to relapse and develop severe symptoms of depression and anxiety again, but they do need to be mindful of what is required to prevent these symptoms from reoccurring, whether that is medication, sleep, exercise, nutrition, or all of the above. Stress in life is inevitable, and a brain that is predisposed to any form of mental illness (depression, anxiety, OCD) needs to be well-nurtured so that it can weather the storms.

Imagine a tree or plant in your yard or on your block somewhere. If it is not watered, fed with sunlight, and cared for, it will easily be blown over in a storm. Our brains work the same way.

The good news? Stress-related depression and anxiety are usually much shorter-lived than a postpartum mood and anxiety disorder like PPD. This is especially true if you have some awareness about what your brain and body need to be well, and you can ask for help early.

With that in mind, here are 10 tips on how to both manage stress when it comes in uninvited and how to take care of yourself so the stress doesn't take over.

1. **Notice when your life speeds up.** Most of us, when life gets busy, speed right up along with it. We tend to push aside our needs when we are in periods of busy-ness, and we end up making very little, if any, time for self-care. We forget to eat. We skip the exercise. We stay up later. We give up our rest, our breaks, and our downtime, because we feel like we have to in order to get things done. But this never works, because more times than not, we end up running out of fuel. Crashing. We forget to put on our own oxygen mask first, and then we have nothing left to give to anyone. So, instead, notice when your life gets fuller and, instead of rushing to meet it, make a conscious effort to slow *yourself* down. Schedule in meals, exercise, sleep, and breaks. In the long run these moments will save you.
2. **Have a mantra.** "*I am okay even when I don't feel that way*," "*This too shall pass*," "*I matter*." This can be anything that helps you remember that you are doing your best, you are not superhuman, and times when you don't feel great do not equate to you not *being* great.
3. **Take care of the cold.** When you notice early signs of emotional distress (tension, headache, belly upset, tearfulness), nourish yourself like you would at the earliest hints of a cold. When you wake up with a sore throat or runny nose, do you rush out for an hour-long workout or stay up as late as you can? Let's hope not. So, let's prevent the flu. Eat your veggies and plenty of protein. Get some rest. Be kind to yourself as you would if you were noticing early signs of physical distress.
4. **Give yourself permission to feel bad.** With changes in weather, hormonal shifts, increased workloads, childcare demands, and household chores piling up, it would be impossible not to feel overwhelmed. Again, remember it is not the feelings of overwhelm that are problematic, but whether you take care of yourself when you notice them.

5. **Talk to someone.** Blog. Go see your therapist. Talk to your partner or best friend or random grocery store clerk who asks you how your day is going. When we hold our tension inside, it will inevitably build up until there is no more room to store it. Give yourself some space.
6. **Breathe.** Seriously. When we are stressed, we all tend to become physically tense and take short, shallow chest breaths. We use only a limited amount of our lung capacity. When we respond physically to an event or situation this way, we tell our brains that it is important to panic. Even if this isn't true. Our brains need adequate oxygen to function effectively, and believe it or not, we have a huge amount of control over this. Practicing deep belly (or diaphragmatic) breathing can literally change our physiological response to stress.
7. **Know that it will pass.** Because it will. Perspective is really important during periods of stress, and it is also the first to go when we become depressed or anxious. And you can remind yourself if this is your mantra: "This Too Shall Pass."
8. **Avoid alcohol, drugs, and caffeine.** It is so easy to drink one too many glasses of wine or coffee when you are feeling bad because, in the moment, it feels like it will help. But the truth is that drugs and alcohol will not help you to feel less depressed (they are depressants), and caffeine will not help you to feel less anxious (it is a stimulant).
9. **Acknowledge cognitive distortions.** This is the basis for cognitive behavioral therapy (CBT), and we know a huge amount about how and why thoughts really do impact the way we feel. Catastrophic thinking, should statements, all-or-nothing thinking, discounting the positives, discounting your coping skills, "what if" thinking, fortune telling, and overestimating the threat will, inevitably, make you feel awful.
10. **Be mindful of your emotional limit.** Often, managing your stress alone just isn't going to cut it. Don't be afraid to call and make an appointment with your therapist again as you may need additional support during this time. Sometimes, just one or two sessions back will be all you need to resurface again.

The Value of Pleasure

Somehow, pleasure has become a bad word. Or a word that brings up a response of *"I don't have time"* or *"That would be nice"* or maybe, even, *"What the hell is that?"* Somehow, in motherhood, finding or engaging in pleasure has become an impossible and seemingly selfish endeavor.

But man, it is an important part of being human.

For the purpose of this discussion, I am going to define pleasure as *an experience of somatic joy. An experience that involves the human senses and physical experience of "feeling good" in our bodies.* Pleasure, quite frankly, does not involve our thinking and our story lines. **Pleasure is, simply, a sensory experience that invokes pleasant sensations.**

I don't just mean sex. Though, of course that is certainly one way to access pleasure.

Engaging in pleasurable activities (think sight, sound, touch, taste, smell) releases dopamine in our brains. This experience of pleasure and reward sets into motion what is called a *pleasure pathway*—the brain remembers that this activity brings pleasure and so then desires more of this activity, knowing that it brings feelings associated with happiness. In other words, the brain begins to make connections between that activity and pleasure, encouraging us to repeat the behavior.

This, of course, can be problematic if the activity we are engaging in is potentially bad for us, like substance use, screen time, or the like. **But what if the activity is actually good for us? What if the activity leads to connections with ourselves, our loved ones, or the world around us?**

Sometimes, in parenthood, we get mashed up in the struggle. The suffering. The pain. Sometimes we truly forget the importance of pleasure.

So, I have an experiment for you to try this week. For the next seven days, I would like you to consider ways to find pleasure throughout your day. Each day, consider little things that might be right in front of you the whole time.

The smell of your baby's head.

The sound of a child's giggle.

The sensation of sun on your face.

The experience of tasting something delicious.

The sensory experience of a tight hug by someone you love.

The physical experience of receiving a shoulder rub, or a foot rub, or someone (maybe a child!) playing with your hair.

The genuine receipt of a compliment.

The feeling of grass under your feet, or the smell of the woods in fall, of the dance of leaves in the breeze, or the taste of the final tomatoes of the season that finally grow red on their vine.

A pet's snuggle.

A delicious cup of tea or coffee in the morning, enjoyed slowly.

A warm bath or a hot shower.

Get the gist?

But here is the thing about it all. In order to experience the pleasure—in order to fully be in your body enough to *feel* the pleasure—you need to slow down. Pleasure is an experience that often passes quickly, and if you don't pause, you will likely miss it.

Along with this experiment comes a guarantee. If you really try this, if you commit to this practice, you will report more happiness at the end of the week. Even when life feels really hard.

Worth the try?

Ten Tips for Getting Through Seasonal Depression

Are you a mom who struggles with the change of seasons? If so, you are not alone. If you saw yourself in the earlier chapter on Seasonal Affective Disorder, then these tips are likely to move you through the darker and colder months.

Transition: movement, passage, or change from one position, state, stage, subject, concept, etc., to another; change: *the transition from adolescence to adulthood.*

Fall is the season of change. The light changes. The temperature changes. The leaves and flowers and last pieces of summer-ness change. School starts. Work might be busier. People are outside less. As we add layers of clothing, many of us also add layers of distress. The start of autumn is exciting for many, but for others, it brings with it a veil of worry, anxiety, sadness, and discomfort in the form of depressed or anxious moods or a period of seasonal depression.

For moms who are already struggling with postpartum depression and/or anxiety, this change can feel like too much to bear. At my office in Boulder, my phone rings more often, and so I can see the connection pretty clearly.

Below are some suggestions about how to take care of yourself if you are one of the many who find your emotional wellness slipping away with the daylight, whether it's full-blown seasonal affective disorder, known as seasonal depression, or a worsening of your moods when fall comes. This is, of course, not a cure-all, or a reason not to seek out face-to-face support if you are really having a tough time, or a way of telling you that if you just tried harder, you would feel better (we all know that postpartum depression and anxiety don't work that way). Rather, consider the 10 tips below to be useful strategies you can pull out as needed to help you get through seasonal depression and the bumps of transition.

1. **Try to identify one thing that remains consistent through this transition, and pay attention to it.** This can be something as literal as "I take a shower every morning," as practice-based as "I take five deep breaths when I notice myself becoming anxious," or as metaphorical as "I am a tree withstanding a storm" or "I am a stone in a raging river." Or, you may want to try identifying, out loud, all of the parts of you that remain steady despite the changes around you: "I am a woman. I live in ___. I am a mother. My baby's name is ____." When we feel ungrounded, it can be reassuring to know that we can count on something.
2. **Make sure you are meeting your basic needs.** Sleep, nutrition (including adequate protein intake), exercise, and water intake are all imperative for brain health and functioning and can help us to better tolerate the effects of stress.

3. **Stay connected.** As the weather changes, we all seem to go back indoors, and too often, this isolation contributes to feelings of depression and anxiety. Reach out to those people in your life whom you feel your best around.
4. **Ask yourself what it is that you need to feel well *today*.** In other words, you can't change the change, but you can make choices around the way you care for yourself during this change. Perhaps you need to ask for more help/support from your partner, family, or friends. Maybe you need a bit more exercise, or more rest. Maybe you need to cut down on your to-do list. What you need now may be different three months from now.
5. **Be kind to yourself.** Yeah, I know. This one can be hard, especially if you are one of the many who has very high expectations of yourself. But the truth is that most people feel the ripple of change, so it makes sense that you may begin to feel a bit unmoored at this time. When you beat yourself up for feeling out of sorts, it adds a whole new level of distress.
6. **Talk about it.** If you give yourself permission to talk about the effect seasonal change is having on you, you will most likely find that others understand and validate how you feel. Company is truly healing.
7. **Plan ahead for the winter months.** Many people suffer from an illness called Seasonal Affective Disorder (SAD) that occurs, most commonly, during winter when the daylight hours are shortest. If you know that you struggle during the winter, you may want to consider thinking ahead so you are prepared to take really good care of yourself when you need it most. If you cook, you may want to consider preparing some healthy meals that can be frozen and reheated when your motivation for cooking is lessoned (or asking friends and family to help you with this!). If you are not currently taking a multivitamin, you may want to consider starting one so that you build up your immunity, your nutritional intake, and your energy levels. Perhaps you can look ahead at finding childcare for times when you crave breaks away from the house, exercise that does not involve being attached to your baby, and/or connecting with a community of friends. Maybe you can preregister for an exercise class at your local rec center. This transition time may be the perfect opportunity to look ahead to what you *might* need to feel well later.
8. **Add color to your home.** This is kind of a materialistic one, I know, but this may be a great time to add color and brightness. Those of us who live in the land of seasons get a burst of color (albeit fall color) and then all of the color in our environment seems to disappear. Recharging your environment may help to keep your spirits up.
9. **Breathe.** Seriously. When we get ramped up in our emotions, we tend to move faster to stay ahead of feelings that are distressing. We do more.

Unfortunately, counter to expectation, this actually can make us feel more anxious. If you notice that you are becoming depressed or anxious during this time, you may find that a few deep belly breaths help to calm the tension ... and slow you down.

10. **Try your best to have perspective.** This is hard when you aren't feeling great, but it is important. Seasons change. Transitions come and go. Those of us who are mothers know that nothing stays around forever ... neither the pleasant (she is sleeping!) nor the unpleasant (he will never stop crying!). To use a very overstated phrase, "this too shall pass." That doesn't mean that this transition will be easy, but it won't last forever. Autumn will come and go, as will winter. Then spring will peak its head out again, and soon we'll be making our way back to summer. We get to do it again, maybe this time with a little more understanding, tolerance, and practice.

Nine Ways to Beat Back the Winter Blues for Moms with Postpartum Depression

Are you a mom who struggles with the change in seasons? If so, you are not alone. If you saw yourself in the earlier chapter on Seasonal Affective Disorder, then these tips are likely to help you to move through the darker and colder months.

1. **If you do see sunlight, try to get outside, even if for only a few moments.** Sunlight and the vitamin D our skin can manufacture when exposed to it can lift the winter blues, and so if you see it, I encourage you to pocket some of it if you can. Or, if it is too cold to be outside, stand or sit by a window and soak up whatever rays are available to you.
2. **Consider a way to get movement and exercise while at home.** Yoga or exercise DVDs can be a great way to bring your movement home to you. Or dance! A mom I have been seeing in my office uses the long winter months to turn up the music she loves and boogie with her baby. If your children are little enough, they might just love the movement, too. And watching you may just be the entertainment your little one needs! Plus, exercise can help with your postpartum depression, too.
3. **Make sure you are taking a high-potency multivitamin and omega-3 supplement.** If fresh fruits and vegetables are at a minimum, do what you can to replenish this necessary brain food.
4. **Replace cold water with warm water with lemon and honey or tea.** While excess fruit juices or other sweetened beverages are not ideal, spicing up your water so that you can get enough is certainly encouraged. Your brain and body need adequate hydration to function efficiently.
5. **Reach out as much as you can for support and company.** Can you enlist the help of friends for meal deliveries or help with your baby? If it feels too hard to get out, consider asking your community to come to you. You are not alone, and you certainly don't need to be. If asking for this help yourself feels too difficult, is there someone who can ask for you?
6. **For more moderate to severe symptoms, reaching out for the support of a trained psychotherapist can be imperative.** To find support near you, check out the Resources section or go to postpartumprogress.com and click on "Find Help" for a list of treatment programs, specialists, and support groups.
7. **For many women who struggle with seasonal affective disorder, medication support can be a valuable part of treatment.** If you have questions or concerns about this, I encourage you to speak with your therapist or care provider.

8. **Bright light therapy has been shown to reduce symptoms of depression in some women.** For women who suffer from both postpartum depression and seasonal affective disorder, this may be a helpful addition to treatment.
9. **Finally, be kind to yourself and notice if you are beating yourself up for feeling down.** You are not alone. Many, many other mothers out there feel similar to the way you do, whether they have seasonal affective disorder, postpartum depression, or both. I promise.

Finding Emotional Balance

We have all heard it many times before: Moms need to take good care of themselves so they can also be strong for their babies and children, and their families. This goes for any mom, whether she is suffering from a postpartum mood and anxiety disorder like postpartum depression or not. But for the 20 percent or so of moms who are in a less resilient and more vulnerable place, this need cannot be repeated enough.

FILL YOURSELVES UP AS BEST YOU CAN.

This is much easier for those women whose mood or anxiety disorder is not severe, but often the support of medication and/or therapy is needed in order to get to the place where the self-caring can even begin. One thing that comes across in all of the research is that brains and bodies are connected intimately. One cannot be healthy without the health and support of the other.

So, with that said, here are some helpful tips and strategies to make sure you are doing what you can for your body and brain during postpartum depression.

1. **Adequate nutrition:** Our brains need healthy nutrition, including protein, to function adequately. In fact, "feel good hormones" such as serotonin are not naturally occurring in our bodies. Instead, we must consume certain amino acids in the food we eat, which our bodies will then use as building blocks to create these hormones. A well-balanced diet with adequate protein intake is required for optimal emotional well-being.

   HOW TO DO THIS: Adequate nutritional intake does not necessarily mean that you need to sit down to three full meals a day, which is not always possible with a newborn. At the grocery store, find a number of healthy, protein-based snacks you can grab on the go, keep in your diaper bag, stash in a desk drawer at work, or place on your bedside table. These might include but are not limited to nuts, nut butters, lean sandwich meats, hard-boiled eggs, yogurt, protein shakes, or protein bars. Be on the lookout for sugar as a main ingredient, however. Make sure the snacks you choose are low in sugar and high in protein. A good sleep tip: Make sure that the last thing you eat at night is protein-based rather than sugar-based. This can help with sleep quality and help prevent frequent waking due to blood sugar shifts during sleep.

2. **Adequate sleep:** While having a newborn certainly does make it difficult to get the same quality and quantity of sleep you achieved before you were a mama, sleep deprivation should be monitored. One recent study showed that quality of sleep is a higher predictor for postpartum depression and anxiety than the temperament of one's baby

(meaning a mom with a difficult baby who gets "enough" sleep is less likely to become depressed/anxious than a mom with an "easy baby" who is sleep deprived) ... and so getting enough sleep cannot be emphasized enough.

HOW TO DO THIS: This one is important for all moms, but especially those who are at high risk for developing a postpartum mood or anxiety disorder. One way to think of this goal is to attempt to get at least five hours of uninterrupted sleep at least three to four nights per week. Those of you whose babies are taking a bottle will have an easier time with this one, I know, but I encourage every mama to shoot for this. Enlist the help of your husband, partner, family member, friend, or hired support. If possible, sleep in a different room for these blocks of sleep; or if this isn't possible, try earplugs or a white noise machine. During the day, do your best to sleep or rest when your baby sleeps.

3. **Mild to moderate exercise:** Women who get some form of mild to moderate exercise each day are generally less likely to become depressed or anxious than those who do not. This does not mean that you have to go to the gym. Or run a marathon. Or even get out to attend a yoga class. What we are referring to here is "movement and activity," which helps to increase endorphins and decrease stress hormones like cortisol.

   HOW TO DO THIS: Walks with your baby, stretching while your baby sleeps or while he/she watches you, vacuuming or other household projects (if you enjoy them), dancing, mild or moderate running, yoga, etc.

4. **Building community:** Inadequate social support is one of the leading factors in developing depression or anxiety postpartum. Community allows for validation, emotional and logistical support, and company.

   HOW TO DO THIS: Have a friend set up a meal train. Join moms groups, group exercise classes, breastfeeding clubs, online blogs or support networks, or couples counseling when needed. Go on date nights (in or outside your home). Tap into your religious or spiritual communities.

5. **Breathe:** When we are stressed or anxious, most of us are not breathing adequately. When we breathe with our full lung capacity, we give our brain the amount of fresh oxygen it needs to function efficiently.

   HOW TO DO THIS: *Diaphragmatic breathing* is the term used to describe full belly breathing. In order to achieve this, place your hand on your lower belly and take a deep breath, attempting to bring that breath all the way down to the part of your belly that makes your hand rise and fall. One way to extend this breath is to also notice the space between your inhale and exhale, and your exhale and inhale. This breath takes practice, so be patient with yourself. You might set the goal of 10 deep belly breaths each day. Over time this may become second nature.

6. **Deep relaxation strategies:** When we are stressed and anxious, we often forget what it feels like to be relaxed. Reminding your body that this is possible is important.

   HOW TO DO THIS: *Progressive relaxation:* In a lying-down or comfortable position, tense and relax each part of your body either from head-to-toe or from toe-to-head. Notice what it feels like to be tense (in your toes, foot, calf, and onward) and then what it feels like to be completely relaxed. When you have gone through each body part in succession, tense and then release your entire body at once. This is often a great tool to use when you're having a hard time falling asleep.

7. **Grounding exercises:** Often, anxiety (including panic) includes a sense of un-groundedness, floating, or ruminating about the pastor future. Reminding yourself to be in the moment can decrease the symptoms that accompany the inability to be present.

HOW TO DO THIS: Notice, and say out loud, where you are in the moment. What do you see? What do you hear? What do you feel? What do you taste? What do you smell? This exercise can take as much or as little time as you have. The goal is simply to bring you back to the moment.

Getting Postpartum Anxiety to Back Off

Postpartum anxiety is probably the most common beast in my office. This big, furry, gnarly clawed beast takes many different shapes—general anxiety, panic, OCD, for example—but usually the annoying, mean, and seemingly relentless monster has a big "A" for anxiety stamped on his forehead. This monster is ferocious at times, making it impossible for moms to sleep, eat, breathe, and think clearly. He is on a serious mission, no doubt. Sometimes he is so big and impending that I get a sense of his foul breath from my chair. Even though it is not me he is chasing, I get a glimpse of what it must feel like to be the mom who is living in his humongous shadow. Not good.

The moms who come into my office in an effort to get the heck out of this guy's path have no idea of how on Earth to do this, or if it's even possible. For these moms, this snaggletoothed misery called postpartum anxiety is all they can see. He makes it this way because he seems to know exactly how to get back into their line of sight when they begin to turn away.

Annoying, to say the least.

So, I thought I'd take a minute to explain, from my chair, what goes into getting postpartum anxiety off your back. So that, if you don't already, you'll have a sense of how you might overpower him. The reality is that he is actually not as strong and lethal as he looks. I know he *feels* strong and invincible—he is really, really skilled at that—but the truth is that he does melt when you throw the right kind of water on him.

When I work with moms who are in battle with postpartum anxiety, I break the treatment down into four parts:

1. Looking at treating the symptoms and managing crises
2. Understanding the role that thoughts play in anxiety
3. Understanding the non-biological causes of the anxiety
4. Learning to tolerate anxiety and distress when it occurs

If you want to stick with the monster metaphor, the four things look like this:

1. Treating his bite
2. Understanding the role that your fear of him plays in his strength
3. Understanding why he is pestering YOU of all people
4. Learning how to be okay even when he is knocking at your door

Four Tips for Reducing Postpartum Anxiety

1. **Treating his bite (or treating the symptoms):** First and foremost, we have got to stop the bleeding, right? If a mom is anxious all of the time and, because of this, unable to meet her body's basic needs, if she is suffering from panic attacks, or if she is having the intrusive thoughts of postpartum OCD, we need to take care of her brain so it can be healthier. For many moms, this will involve medication because, truthfully, when these things happen, it lets us know that your brain is sick and needs to become more resilient. SSRI medication (like Zoloft) and benzodiazepines (like Klonopin) are usually very, very helpful in this (and also known to be safe for breastfeeding moms, by the way).

   We also know that things like sleep, healthy nutrition (especially adequate protein intake because amino acids found in proteins are building blocks to serotonin, the feel-good hormone in the brain), water, and oxygen are important in brain health. So I always have conversations with my client moms about how to make sure they are getting these things. Help at night and/or other strategies for sleep as well as protein-based snacks and water in her diaper bag, car, bedside table, and desk at work are imperative. As is learning how to breathe effectively. Did you know that when we are anxious, we are usually breathing in our chest and actually using only about a third of our lung capacity? Think hyperventilation to the extreme. In order for our brains to settle rather than react, they need enough oxygen. The moms whom I see get a lesson or 20 on how to take a deep diaphragmatic (or belly) breath because this will literally change their physiological reactions to stress. Exercise also helps the brain to be strong, as it has been shown to lower cortisol levels in folks who do it.

2. **Understanding the role that your fear of this monster plays in its strength (or understanding the role that thoughts play in postpartum anxiety):** Anxiety, like monsters, loves when you are afraid. Anxiety gets more power from this fear; it seems to increase tremendously when you are afraid of being anxious, afraid of having a panic attack, or afraid of the power that your intrusive thoughts have. This is the basis for cognitive behavioral therapy (CBT), and there is a huge amount of research on the positive effects that CBT has on pregnant and postpartum moms who are anxious.

   In my office, I use cognitive therapy components often, teaching moms how to identify negative thoughts (such as the "shoulds," all-or-nothing thinking, catastrophic thinking, discounting the positives, overestimating the threat, "what-if" thinking, and over-generalization) and helping them learn to replace these thoughts with something more useful (and true). What these moms find is that when they take away the nourishment for that big, bad monster, he begins to get weaker. He may still be around when all is said and done, but more times than not he is shaking at the knees. There is a great book, by the way, that helps moms to use these techniques called *The Pregnancy and Postpartum Anxiety Workbook,* by Pamela Wiegartz and Kevin Gyoerkoe.

3. **Understanding why he is pestering YOU of all people (or understanding the non-biological causes of the anxiety):** We know that anxiety is a physiological response to a stressful event and that symptoms like elevated heart rate, shallow breathing, dizziness, and sweaty palms are all physical responses to hormones (like cortisol) that are released in the limbic brain.

   But what, exactly, is triggering this brain reaction? Sometimes there may be no apparent cause. Often moms will say that "on paper everything is going well" and anxiety (that darned monster) just lingers anyway. Usually, though, something is being triggered that causes the brain to assume it needs to panic. Does your crying baby remind you of a time when your needs were not met? Does the reality of being responsible for a baby stir up memories of needing to be overly responsible as a child? Do you hold expectations of yourself in motherhood that are unrealistic and provided by people and books rather than yourself? Has the shift in becoming a mom created identity changes that feel unfamiliar (and therefore disconcerting) to you?

   Once we understand *why* we feel so anxious, we can begin the process of validating and empathizing with ourselves because *of course* we would be feeling anxious given many of the triggers that motherhood initiates. Once you get why that big guy is following YOU around, you just might be able to forgive him a bit. Want him to stay? Definitely not, but understand his crush? Perhaps.

4. **Learning how to be okay when he is knocking at your door (or learning to tolerate postpartum anxiety and distress when it occurs):** The truth is, folks, that if those of us who treat postpartum depression and anxiety told moms we were *curing* them of their anxiety, we would be setting them up for disappointment. Being a mom is overwhelming, and it is, at a certain level, entirely normal and appropriate for moms to be anxious from time to time.

   What is not normal or appropriate is for moms to be anxious *all* the time or for anxiety to interfere with daily life. When this happens, it tells us that something else is going on outside of the normal strains of being a mama. For moms who suffer from an anxiety disorder, any level of anxiety becomes distressing because they have learned that anxiety is dangerous. So, we need to teach moms how to know that they will be okay even when they feel this way.

> This does not mean, by the way, that moms need to ignore the anxiety, push it away, or pretend it doesn't exist; this would be no more possible (or helpful) than telling your ears not to hear the loud banging at the back door. But what I do focus on in my office is helping moms learn to acknowledge their anxiety at the lowest level that it exists, give themselves a big, huge hug around the fact that they are feeling anxious (usually for very good reason, even if it is just the fact that they are caring for a little, tiny person) rather than judge themselves for it, and then take super-duper good care of themselves in that moment so their anxiety rests (take some deep breaths, eat something protein-based, go for a walk, call a friend, take a break, etc.). We actually don't need to fix anxiety every time it comes up, but what we can do is acknowledge it, understand it, and then be really, really kind to ourselves.

None of this is easy. Often, it takes an army to fight off this unrelenting beast. But it is possible, even when it feels like it is not.

Why Mindfulness Matters

Have you ever had one of those weeks in which each moment of each day has felt like playing catch-up? When I'm having one of these weeks, I find myself exhausted upon waking up, harried through breakfast with my kids, late for preschool drop-off, barely on time for my first client session of the day, behind on paperwork, late for pickup, short-tempered through dinner and bath time, impatient during book time before bed, too lazy to eat anything other than cereal for dinner, and then exhausted again at bedtime. All that is not including the time I've spent keeping the house in some kind of order, paying my bills, folding laundry that has been sitting in the laundry room for days, supporting friends who just had babies, staying connected to my husband, playing with my daughters, and, if I am lucky, getting to yoga.

When I have one of these weeks, I sometimes laugh to myself when I think about how people often assume that since I am a specialist in the field of mental health and perinatal mood disorders, I've figured it all out. That I've got it down. That I am somehow superhuman.

Wouldn't that be nice?

You see, we are all human. We all have to practice being the best that we can be. We all have these weeks, no matter how much we love our children or our jobs or our friends. We all survive.

When I do make it to my yoga class, I'm reminded of what's important during hectic weeks like these as well as in any time of stress: mindfulness. While these times of stress may seem infinite when struggling with PPD or another perinatal mood or anxiety disorder, stress will still show up from time to time after you have recovered.

So I invite you, just for a moment, to step onto your "mat"—in whatever way that "mat" presents itself to you:

Close your eyes. Yes, if you feel safe enough to close them for just a moment. Notice your breath. Are you breathing quickly? Shallowly? Not at all? Slow it down. Bring that breath all the way to the bottom of your belly. Notice for one brief moment the space between your inhale and your exhale.

Then, become aware of your surroundings. What do you hear? What does it feel like to be sitting in your chair or on your mat? What does it feel like to be "you" right this second, and in all of your complicated glory? What does it feel like to be you without all of the self-judgment but simply just the way that you are? Oh, and don't forget about your breath.

In one of my yoga classes, the teacher spoke about how what happens on the yoga mat is a perfect reflection of what happens in our lives outside of the yoga studio. Do we rush through postures? Do we forget to breathe? Are we judging ourselves and becoming frustrated when we can't get into a certain pose or aren't "good enough" at yoga? Are we comparing ourselves to the others in the room? Are we paying attention to what feels right in our bodies, or are we doing what we think our bodies "should" do and therefore putting ourselves at risk for injury? What happens when we exist in these ways in a yoga class? We lose our balance. We fall. We become more frustrated.

Instead, what would happen if we decided to slow down? To breathe. Deeply. To pay attention to what feels right today, not yesterday or tomorrow, but today at this very instant? What would happen if we chose to look inside rather than around the room at others? If we decided to give our bodies and ourselves the benefit of the doubt?

I'll tell you: We would balance.

You see, it's a common tendency to speed up when we become stressed or overwhelmed. We try to cram more in so we can feel more accomplished. We try to push ourselves because we feel like we should, and we become tired and depleted in the doing. When we are stressed, most of us speak in ways that are unkind to ourselves, judgmental, and very non-empathetic. "I can't believe you can't do this," we say. "You are so lame for being such a failure and for falling behind," we criticize. "Obviously you will never be able to do it," we command. Usually, we forget to breathe. And we lose our balance.

However, the more mindful we are, the more grounded we become. When we move and make choices with intention, we are rewarded with calm more often than not. Being a mama is hard, and we are pushed and moved in more ways than we can count. Add a perinatal mood or anxiety disorder, and we can feel more off-balance than ever.

Practicing mindfulness does not have to happen in a yoga studio or even on a real-life yoga mat. It can happen anywhere. Sometimes it takes practice, but it is most certainly worth the try.

A Tool Kit for Postpartum Anxiety and Panic Symptoms

The term *postpartum depression* can be a disservice to many, many women who struggle during pregnancy and/or postpartum. Many of these women don't reach out for help because, well, they are not necessarily depressed and so therefore assume that their struggle is not with postpartum depression.

In fact, the most common symptom of postpartum depression is not sadness at all: It is anxiety and agitation. While many women who struggle might have periods of sadness, depression, and tearfulness, the overwhelming symptoms that cause them great pain are difficulty concentrating, excessive worry, high-level overwhelm, racing thoughts, and difficulty sleeping.

Many of these women will suffer from a varying degree of panic, and anxiety attacks are not uncommon (or perhaps they will have postpartum anxiety or OCD).

So, what is this all about, and what can be done in the moment to alleviate some of the fear that comes along with these symptoms? Understandably, moms often want an answer to "Why is this happening to me? What is causing this?" As always, this is a question that doesn't necessarily come with one quick answer as each woman has a unique set of circumstances that might be playing a part. But we do have ideas of what may be at issue here. Fortunately, there are a number of strategies that are known to work well and alleviate some of the symptoms of mild to moderate anxiety. Before we get to those, let's take a closer look at some of the things that might be causing these symptoms.

1. **Brain chemistry imbalance:** High-level anxiety (including postpartum OCD) is often caused by imbalances in the "feel good" chemicals in our brains. Serotonin, dopamine, and norepinephrine are the neurotransmitters that are responsible for emotional balance, and sudden drops in hormones postpartum are believed to have a direct impact on the functioning of these important systems of the brain. Antidepressant medications such as SSRIs (including but not limited to Zoloft) have been shown to work effectively at reducing symptoms of anxiety in the postpartum period (usually a woman will notice a reduction in symptoms two to three weeks after starting a medication). Many of these medications have been shown to be safe during pregnancy and while breastfeeding. Benzodiazepines (including but not limited to Xanax) have been shown to work effectively at reducing symptoms associated with panic attacks and high-level anxiety (often in conjunction with an SSRI). While it is recommended that women not cease using a benzodiazepine during pregnancy or breastfeeding if her symptoms are severe and/or if she has benefited from them prior to her pregnancy, some of these medications have a small risk to infants, so careful monitoring by a physician

is important. For women whose anxiety is severe, the recommended treatment is medication along with psychotherapy.

2. **Negative thought patterns:** Oh, the many changes that occur when a baby is born! Women who are worriers, who are perfectionists, who have high and often unrealistic expectations for themselves, or who have a tendency toward negative thinking prior to becoming pregnant are at risk of developing more severe postpartum anxiety once a baby is born. For these women, the new lack of control, many responsibilities of parenting, and reality of caring for a newborn all contribute to racing thoughts and heightened worry. Psychotherapy is an important part of the treatment for these women. Cognitive behavioral therapy (CBT), mindfulness, stress reduction strategies, work around identity shifting, and early trauma history processing (if it exists) have all been effectively supported through psychotherapeutic work with a trained professional.
3. **Nutrient depletion:** Numerous studies have linked nutrient depletion during pregnancy and postpartum to depression and anxiety in many mothers. The role of healthy eating and monitored vitamin supplements, if/when necessary, cannot be underestimated in moms' health and wellness. Even women who think they are eating a balanced diet may not be replenishing themselves enough after childbirth and breastfeeding to facilitate the production of serotonin and the balance of blood sugar. Often, symptoms such as agitation, shakiness, foggy-headedness, and nervousness can be linked to hunger and poor eating habits in many women.
4. **Sleep deprivation:** Yes, I know: Having a newborn drastically limits the time that all moms spend asleep. Frequent night waking, breastfeeding, and high anxiety make it difficult for most moms to get the rest they need for optimum health. But here is the thing: Moms who are moderately or severely anxious are usually also moms who report getting less than four hours of uninterrupted sleep a night. When these moms increase their sleep time through medication, strategy building, and/or relaxation techniques, their anxiety symptoms often decrease.
5. **Dehydration:** Some studies have suggested that dehydration contributes to anxiety symptoms, including jumpiness and agitation. Moms, especially those who are breastfeeding, are often not drinking adequate amounts of water (at least eight 8-ounce glasses of water a day or more). Proper water consumption is necessary for efficient transportation of the hormones and neurotransmitters required for balanced emotion.
6. **Pregnancy-related physical ailments and insufficient breathing:** Most women who feel anxious will notice that their breathing is shallow. Whether

this is because a pregnant mom's diaphragm is being squished by her growing baby or because she is simply not focused on the length and quality of her breath, a lack of sufficient oxygen to the brain leads to dizziness, further shortness of breath, light-headedness, and elevated heart rate. Often, focused and mindful breath work will noticeably reduce these symptoms.

So ... now for that tool kit. You know, the one you need by your side if and when you begin to notice the early signs of anxiety and/or panic emerge.

1. Take 10 deep belly breaths (also known as diaphragmatic breathing).
2. Drink a big glass of water.
3. Eat a protein-based snack such as lean meats, nuts, cheese, or a hard-boiled egg.
4. Ground yourself in the present: Look around you and note (out loud if possible) everything that you can access in all five senses. What do you see? What can you hear? What do you smell? What does it feel like to be sitting on your chair? What, exactly, do you taste as you eat your snack?
5. Find a "mantra" of sorts that you can tell yourself, such as "I am going to be okay," "I am doing the best I can," or "I am taking care of myself."
6. Go outside. Stretch. Feel yourself move and notice the sensations in your body.
7. Once your initial symptoms decrease, find some help so you can take a nap and get the rest you need.
8. If need be, call your therapist, your doctor, or someone you trust to come and be with you until you feel better.

When the Risk of Not Getting Help for PPD Just Isn't Worth It

Babies are resilient. We know this to be true. But babies and children may be negatively impacted by a mom's untreated depression, anxiety, or other mood disorder during pregnancy or postpartum. It seems to me this might not be a risk worth taking. Moms need help for PPD.

Please carefully note the specifics of what I said above: "Babies and children may be negatively impacted by a mother's **untreated** depression, anxiety, or other mood disorder during pregnancy or postpartum." Many, many of you can attest to the fact that children whose mothers suffered from prenatal or postpartum depression or anxiety and received treatment are just fine—even thriving.

Moms who make it a priority to get help for PPD, follow treatment recommendations from a trained professional, get well, and take care of themselves do so to benefit not just themselves but also their children. Most of these kiddos go on to be happy and healthy preschoolers, teens, and adults.

We worry when a mom's depression or anxiety goes untreated. In these instances, emotional, social, and developmental delays in babies and children can occur. I say this fully knowing that this fact may bring additional layers of anxiety to women who already suffer, and I am hopeful that those women understand that this statement is not a condemnation or a finger shake. It is, instead, a compassionate offering through a realistic look at the risks that may come to those who do not reach out for the support they deserve.

Scientists have done some fascinating research on depression in preschoolers. While we know that many factors contribute to the development of depressive symptoms in children this young, and that often these children do not have parents who are depressed themselves (and, conversely, having a depressed parent does not necessarily mean that a young child will also be depressed), we do know that many of these little people may not have received the empathetic attunement and emotional mirroring from their mothers that they need to thrive. Babies need to be attended to and heard, they need to be held and comforted, they desire eye contact and voice recognition, and if a mother is unable to provide these things because she is depressed or anxious, a baby may suffer the consequences.

So, here are some of the risks for babies and children whose mothers suffer from **untreated** prenatal or postpartum depression and anxiety:

- Pregnant women who are depressed are less likely to take adequate care of themselves and their unborn babies.
- Preterm labor has been linked to depression and anxiety in pregnant mothers.

- Preeclampsia has been linked to depression and anxiety in pregnant mothers.
- Depression and anxiety during pregnancy have been linked to low birth weight in babies.
- Babies whose mothers were depressed or anxious during pregnancy are more likely to have eating and sleeping challenges and are more likely to be difficult to soothe.
- Attachment and bonding may be negatively affected, and this can have an impact on a child's ability to form healthy relationships during school-aged years and on through adulthood.
- Fathers whose partners are depressed are also more likely to develop depressive symptoms in the postpartum period. If this happens, neither parent may be able to attend to the emotional needs of their newborn.
- Mothers who have postpartum depression tend to spend less time engaging in eye contact, mirroring facial and voice expressions, and casually playing with their babies. All of these activities are important for bonding and attachment.

With this said, we know that other caregivers, such as a father, grandparent, other family member, friends, and nannies can provide the emotional reciprocity that is needed if and when a mom is temporarily unable. While a baby needs its mother first and foremost, that child will absolutely be okay if, temporarily, it is getting all of its physical and emotional needs met by someone else. What matters most, truly, is that mom gets the support she needs to feel well so she can care for her babe in the ways that are important to both of them.

So, moms, if you are suffering, please get help. For you and for your little one.

Finding Balance between Body, Mind, and Social Network during Postpartum Depression

The "being" and "doing" is a tricky balance that needs to be considered all along the journey toward health and wellness in motherhood. Sometimes you may need to allow yourself to slow down the pace and to acknowledge, once again, where you are and how you are feeling.

We know that perinatal mood and anxiety disorders like postpartum depression are a *biopsychosocial* challenge for women, meaning that they are most likely caused by disruptions or challenges in a woman's biology (physiological system), psychology (emotional and psychological system), and social network (including friends, family, and community). Usually, finding wellness requires a look into all of these areas to see where these strengths and challenges lie. These systems are usually somewhat overlapping, like a Venn diagram. Strength in one area might allow for strength in the other, and vice versa. But wellness almost always involves feelings of wholeness in each of these three areas.

In my practice I often walk women through each one of these areas in an effort to take inventory, so to speak. We look at where she is grounded and full and also where she is feeling untethered and lacking.

The process looks something like this:

PHYSICAL SELF

What are you doing right now to help your physical body to feel strong? What does your nutrition intake look like? How is your sleep? Are you currently taking medication for your postpartum depression or anxiety symptoms, and if not, is it important to have a medication evaluation? Are you pushing yourself too hard? Are you engaging in some exercise each day, whether it's stretching or walking or other more moderate forms? Are you breathing deeply? Are you drinking plenty of water? Are you getting outside to breathe fresh air and feel the sun on your face?

PSYCHOLOGICAL SELF

Are you meeting yourself where you are, or do you need to set more realistic expectations? Are your priorities clear? Are you consumed by the "shoulds" placed on us by society, books, family, and friends, or are you allowing yourself to follow a path that feels right to you? Are you using words of kindness and compassion with yourself, or are you using a tone with yourself that is harsh and unsupportive? Are you engaging in thought patterns that are useful and realistic, or are you engaging in perfectionist thinking? Do you find yourself thinking in black-and-white extremes, or are you allowing yourself to be open to all that is in between? Are old family patterns or unresolved family conflict interfering with your ability to be present with your baby right now? Do you have a trauma history that is resurfacing and deserves attention? Do you have a number of stress reduction and grounding strategies that are useful in times of chaos, or are you feeling ill equipped in this area? Are you currently working with a trained therapist who can help support you and work with you to find new ways of thinking and managing your stress, or is it time for you to find one?

SOCIAL SELF

How supported are you? Are you able to ask for help when you need it? Do you have a community of friends, family, neighbors, and/or health providers to support you along this journey through postpartum depression? Are you and your partner able to work together during this time of high vulnerability, or can you use some support around relationships?

Sometimes it is helpful to see all of this on paper by creating a rough table along the way. If this resonates and if you choose to go this route, you might consider a table in which the horizontal rows list the three areas of wellness (physical, psychological, and social) and the vertical columns provide space for strengths and challenges.

WELLNESS ELEMENT	CURRENT ACTIVITIES SUPPORTING WELLNESS	IS ANYTHING MISSING?
PHYSICAL		
EMOTIONAL/ PSYCHOLOGICAL		
SOCIAL		

I want to reiterate *that this exercise can be confusing and of*ten requires the help of a trained professional who can work with you to sort through the many layers of your being. Sometimes, *sometimes*, simply going through this process with intention can help you to feel more empowered and in control of your wellness. Often, this is not the case, and unbalanced biochemistry or sleep deprivation is just making it too darn difficult to do what you know you need to do to feel better. It is likely that once you find some sense of wholeness and wellness in your physical body (including adequate sleep, nutrition, and balanced biochemistry), the other two areas will be easier to address. Usually, when you feel a bit more whole in all three areas of holistic health, you will feel happy to greet yourself right where you are. You will find joy in simply "being."

Growing is Uncomfortable

I can tell you this for sure: Motherhood is chronically uncomfortable.

No mother anywhere has mastered the feat of being constantly comfortable in motherhood. Some women might believe that the purpose of life is to be comfortable—to create a life that avoids discomfort and pain and that celebrates safety and security. But these women are still working really, really hard to meet this goal and are undeniably increasing their own discomfort in the process.

Because this is not possible. Motherhood is messy. We are being challenged at our core every step of the way. We worry and we are uncertain and we don't know what the heck we are doing most of the time.

Imagine this: Two concentric circles. **The small one in the center is your safety or comfort zone.** Many of us build tall, thick walls around ourselves in an effort to stay in this zone, all cozy and protected. **The outer circle, very large, is your danger zone.** Many of us feel deep threat in this zone, experiencing panic and fight/flight/freeze responses. In this world, we jump back and forth from safety/comfort to danger/risk, and over time our comfort zone becomes smaller while our danger zone becomes larger. Neither of these two zones serves us. **In our comfort zone we are stagnant and bored and unfulfilled and often feel trapped. In our danger zone we are defensive and protective and full of fear.**

Safety zone: We often feel trapped, tight, guarded. Our thoughts are filled with *"I should"* and *"I shouldn't."*

Danger zone: We often feel ungrounded, confused, tense, and defensive. Our thoughts are filled with *"I can't"* and *"What if."*

But, in another world, the one we want to exist in, a circle exists around the safety/comfort zone that is our "growth zone." When we exist in our growth zone, we are uncomfortable, but not in a state of fight/flight/freeze. We have a sense of anticipation but not panic. It is in this zone that we learn and grow and change. We want to live in this zone as often as possible. We *rest* in our safety/comfort zone, and we *strive to live* in our growth zone. **Important note:** We want to be mindful about entering the danger zone because this place is never useful to us. So, in order to remain in a place of growth and not go into a place of danger, we must have boundaries. We must learn how to say no and take care of ourselves so that we don't cross over that fine line. This. Takes. Practice.

Growth zone: We often feel anticipation and uncertainty. We notice physical discomfort, but we are still engaged. Our thoughts are filled with "I can" and "I trust." We may feel fear, but we also feel confidence. In every growth zone there is discomfort. If you are feeling *comfortable*, you are not in this zone.

Okay. Are you following?

So, this week:

Draw three concentric circles.

In the smallest circle, consider what choices you make that are *comfortable and safe* **for you.** Remember, this zone is not bad or problematic, as long as you are using it for rest and repair and not defaulting to this place without intention. *(EXAMPLE: I am lonely and am really craving more friends, but I am somewhat socially uncomfortable. It is just easier to stay at home and not put myself out there.)*

In the largest circle, consider what choices you make that are *dangerous and a risk* **to your mental and/or physical health.** Are you pushing yourself too much and expecting things that are not realistic for you? *(EXAMPLE: I am lonely and want more friends, so I am going to say yes to that invitation to the large gathering in which I know nobody.)*

In the middle circle, consider what choices you make that create opportunities for new things and can fit inside that *growth zone.* Can you push yourself enough to grow and learn without putting yourself in a situation that feels too overwhelming? *(EXAMPLE: I am lonely and want more friends. I am going to say yes to that invitation to walk with some of the other parents from school drop-off, even though I am uncomfortable.)*

The opportunities for growth are endless: communicating needs, learning a new skill, returning to work, bringing in more play/fun/joy, quitting a bad habit, developing a new habit, and so much more.

I believe in you.

Some Strategies for Stress Reduction

Being a mom can be a stressful feat. We are pushed and pulled and twisted by both internal and external stressors, and for all of us, there are times when we feel like we just might crack. Many moms who are struggling with a postpartum mood or anxiety disorder are in this place of high stress more often than not, and these moments can feel way outside of any resemblance of "control." It is likely that these moments are filled with reactions that are based on a need to release pent-up energy that is swirling with anger, agitation, lack of patience, and extreme fatigue. It is in these instances that we are likely to act in ways we wish we hadn't: We yell, we storm out of a room, we crumble in tears of defeat, we close off entirely. In other words, we "react" rather than "respond." You know where these reactions lead us: to more self-judgment and continued vulnerability.

We know of several factors that can be helpful in reducing symptoms of depression and anxiety during pregnancy and the postpartum period:

1. Getting adequate sleep
2. Getting appropriate nutrition
3. Receiving adequate community support
4. Getting mild to moderate daily exercise
5. Having established stress reduction strategies

Usually, moms will have some idea of what the first four elements of emotional wellness involve, and they can picture what it might look like (even if, at the moment, these things seem impossible). But when I discuss the last point with the moms I work with, what I get most of the time is a look of confusion. You see, many of us have learned to cope with stress by reacting in the moment without realizing that we can do so much before the moment becomes too big for us.

So here are several strategies that have been proven to work in slowing down the stress reaction, in creating space for thoughtful responses, and for literally calming the body's response to chaos. It is worth practicing each of these when you need them least—so that they are accessible to you when you need them most.

1. **Diaphragmatic breathing:** When most of us are stressed, we will realize that our breath is short and is contained in the chest. It is as if we literally forget to breathe. Lowered oxygen in the brain can add to physiological reactions that make us feel even more anxious and less clearheaded. Instead, practice the following: Take 10 deep belly breaths, all the way to the bottom of your belly, known as diaphragmatic breathing. Make these breaths as deep and slow as you can. Visualize your belly rising and falling with each breath. If you like,

see if you can notice the space between the inhale and the exhale. After 10 of these breaths, notice how you feel different.

2. **Progressive relaxation:** This is a great practice for when you are in bed at night, especially if you are having a difficult time falling asleep. Most of us, when we are stressed, are holding tension in our bodies, whether it's in our shoulders, neck, or someplace else. We grow accustomed to this tension. Beginning at your feet and working your way up your body to your head, tense up and then relax each part of your body. Your feet, your calves, your entire leg, your buttocks and your hips, your belly and your back, and on and on. Each time you relax a part of your body, notice how this feels. Once you have moved through your whole body, see if you can let go of any remaining tension. Notice how this changes how you feel both internally and externally (when they've practiced this technique enough, moms I work with say that they are asleep before they make it through each body part!).
3. **Visualize a calm and healing place:** This might be a place that you have been before or one that you create in your imagination. This is a place that should feel calm to you— that represents the way you want to feel when you feel the most tense and out of control. As you "create" this place, make sure that you gain access to each sense: What does this place look like? What noises do you hear? Do you smell anything? What does it feel like to be there? Again, the point is to practice "going" to this place when you don't really need it so that, when you do, you can arrive at this place relatively quickly. This exercise acts as a reminder of your ability to feel calm despite the chaos that may exist in the moment.
4. **Ground yourself in the present:** Feelings of anxiety and panic typically involve being focused on the past or the future rather than what is happening in the present moment. If you begin to feel that you are becoming untethered, try the following: Go through each of your five senses and tell yourself, preferably out loud, what is happening. What do you see at this moment? What do you hear? What do you smell? What do you taste? What does it feel like to be sitting in your chair or standing where you are? Do you feel sunlight on your face? Wind in your hair? This exercise reminds you to be here, now.
5. **Brain dump it:** While the first four strategies are about "being," this last is a strategy that involves "doing." Often, high stress involves lots of obsessive thinking and overwhelming thought that can contribute to emotional turbulence. These thoughts get stored in our minds and can make us feel foggy-headed, headachy, or simply unable to think clearly. Sometimes, the simple act of getting onto paper what is flooding your mind is an incredibly

useful tool. Many of the moms I work with will have a pad of paper or a journal by their bed where they can "dump" all of their stress-inducing thoughts. It is likely that this act will clear out some space in your brain for more useful thoughts, and sometimes when you see on paper what has been taking up such space, you may have more of a say in whether or not to let some of it go.

Wishing you some stress relief, Dear Readers.

Six Words That Will Settle Your Nervous System Instantly

Over the course of history, we humans have been taught to strive for more to become better. *More efficient, more skilled, more competent, more thin, more beautiful, more creative, more brave.* Because our brains are wired to think in all-or-nothing ways, we are quick to compare, to feel less than, and to assume that if we aren't that (whatever that must be), then something must be wrong—with us, with the situation, or with the people around us. **In other words, we are pretty quick to assume that a problem exists that needs to be fixed.**

For most of us, "problem" means "threat."

It is important to know that our physiology—our body—does not know the difference between real and perceived threat. For so many of us, the moment we tell ourselves there is a problem is the moment that our bodies go into fight or flight: Our hearts race, we become short of breath, our tummies tighten, and we suddenly don't think very clearly. This is our body's job: to get ready to protect us when we are in danger.

Your baby is crying and you aren't sure why. You burn dinner. A friend doesn't call back when anticipated. Someone disagrees with you about something. You don't feel like playing with your toddler. You are feeling cranky and tired. Your child/children are cranky and tired. Your partner is cranky and tired. You don't feel an instantaneous rush of emotion when you lay eyes on your baby for the first time. Your birth doesn't go as planned. You want or need to stop breastfeeding. Your preteen is, you know, preteening.

These things will, of course, bring up feelings and emotions such as sadness, worry, frustration, or disappointment. But feeling emotion is not a threat. For each of the situations above, support might be necessary. **But none of these examples above, nor many others, are actual threats to our safety.**

So, what are the **six** words that will settle your nervous system instantly?

WHAT. IF. THERE. WAS. NO. PROBLEM?

It's a very important question: **What if this thing that is happening or has happened is not a problem?** It may be inconvenient or uncomfortable, but what if there really is no problem that needs to be fixed or that we need to protect ourselves from? If this were the case, how would you feel? What would you do differently?

Postpartum Depression Recovery: A Therapist's Perspective

Recovery from postpartum depression is so much easier said from my chair than done. I know this. Each time a mom comes into my office for the first time asking if she will ever get better, I am reminded of this very simple truth: It is easy for me to say yes. And yet, I give the same answer many times throughout the treatment process. "Postpartum mood disorders are absolutely treatable. Suffering moms who reach out, accept support, and follow treatment recommendations by trained professionals do see the light at the end of the tunnel."

This reassurance always brings hope. For a while. These moms can breathe again. A smile amidst tears of frustration. Then, after a session or two, these women realize that the work ahead of them is hard. Sometimes, you see, it is almost easier to suffer than it is to think through the pieces that are required for improvement:

Is it okay for me to talk about what I have been feeling? What if this person thinks I am a terrible mother for having these thoughts? Do I take the meds? What do I really need to feel better? Get more sleep? In what reality? Be more thoughtful about what I eat? In what lifetime? Do I really need to revisit the impact that old family conflict or early trauma has had on me now? Where can I find community, and how in the world do I muster the energy and courage to meet other new moms when I am feeling this way? What are the ways that my marriage or partnership needs work? How can I communicate my needs to others with more clarity? And, truthfully, is it even okay for me to do this? I shouldn't really even have needs—I SHOULD be able to do this on my own! How can I make time for myself? What would I do with that time if I had it? And, really, who am I anyway? Where did I go? How will I be able to do this mothering thing without a road map? What do I want my own mothering to look like? What do I want to incorporate from my own childhood, and what do I want to leave behind? Is that even possible, or okay? Practice stress management skills? With what time? Change my thought patterns through cognitive behavioral strategies? With what energy?

Yes. Without a doubt it can feel easier for these moms to suffer in silence. The road to recovery can feel long, overwhelming, hilly, and complicated. And while making that first call is often the hardest first step, the work that is required to get better can feel like a close second. And then that signature "three steps forward, two steps back" rhythm of recovery can feel like a whammy. Yes, my job in this therapy partnership is most certainly easier.

So these moms arrive at my psychotherapy office, some early in their postpartum experience and others having suffered for months or years without yet reaching out. While they wonder if I judge them for their experience and while they worry that I will see them unfit for motherhood, I am always moved by their bravery and their dedication to themselves and their children. They have arrived here and they want to get well. From where I sit, this simple act makes each one of these women absolutely fit for motherhood.

And man, oh man, do I learn from these women! These women are professors. They are artists. They are lawyers, athletes, students, or cooks. Some are writers. Others are labor and delivery nurses. They are pediatricians, obstetricians, accountants, or managers. They are gardeners. They are dedicated mothers. They are wives, partners, and friends. They are human. They are creative. They are witty and wise. These women are thinkers. They are dreamers. They love to laugh. They often cry. These women are bold. They are brave. And they are beautiful.

Yet, each of these women feels about the size of a flea. Or as if she is floating aimlessly. Or that she is worthless in one way or another. And always that she is unable to do this mothering thing as well as everyone else can. Each one of these women feels totally ripped off and caught off guard by her postpartum experience.

"Why can't I do it like all those other women?" they ask.

"All those other women have appointments in my office later today," I answer. Because the truth is that most moms struggle and need support in one way or another, no matter how put together they look on the outside.

What amazes me most about the women I work with is that underneath the chaos of biochemistry imbalance, relationship strife, negative thinking patterns, sleep deprivation, and self-care deprivation, each one of these women really does know what she needs to be well again. It is hard to access this—I know that this is another one of those *easier said than done* moments but I truly believe that the women I see each day are their own experts. These women know better than anyone what they need to feel whole again. My job is to simply ask the right questions. To begin to help connect the dots. To educate, inform, and explore so that these women can understand the pieces that may be contributing to their emotional vulnerabilities.

I'll tell you something. It gets easier for each of them. Over time the "three steps forward" become seven, and the tears are replaced by laughter. Over time the stories of "good mom moments" far outweigh those that are plagued by guilt. Over time these women stand a bit straighter, look a bit more rested, give themselves a bit more permission to be human. While the work may have been the most challenging opportunity yet, they are more of themselves for it. They are more whole. They have a lot more to give to their little ones, whether this be energy, patience, presence, or stress reduction skills.

Then, one day, the women who stick through the hard work walk into my office and declare that they don't feel the need to come in regularly anymore, that they feel ready to take on the roller-coaster ride of motherhood without my regular support. These days are mixed blessings for me. I will miss being a witness on this ride with each of them. Yet the triumph that follows each one of these hard-working women out my door for the last time is moving beyond words.

The Impossible Simplicity of Treating Postpartum Depression

Is it even possible to say that the treatment of postpartum depression and other perinatal mood and anxiety disorders is "simple"? Of course, it doesn't feel that way. For many, many women, getting over and through the challenges of a pre- or postpartum mood disorder such as PPD can feel unfairly complicated. In many ways, it is. We know PPD to be a complex illness, with roots in imbalances and disturbances that cross a woman's physical, social, and psychological being.

But, what if we were to think of the treatment of and recovery from postpartum depression in its most simple form? Would this be helpful?

In my Boulder, Colorado, private psychotherapy practice, I get asked often—*always*, really—about how long recovery from PPD takes. Of course I don't have one answer for this as each mom's challenges and experiences are unique. But sometimes, looking at treatment and recovery as somewhat linear and specific can bring some hope and optimism at a time when it feels that both of these gems are lacking.

So, here goes: What would a map of PPD treatment and recovery look like? What are some things that every mom can consider in working her way toward a stronger sense of well-being?

Again, we know that these illnesses stem from disruptions in a woman's biology, psychology, and social systems, so if we pull these three areas apart and look at each separately, we may be able to make some sense out of a very overwhelming situation.

Where are you being filled up in these areas? Where can you use additional support?

Biology or Physical Body: This is usually the first place to start. Making sure that you are getting your basic needs met is critical in your recovery. Hormone shifts post-delivery that affect biochemistry put every childbearing woman at risk. Add sleep deprivation, nutrient depletion, and possibly a personal or family history of depression, anxiety, or other mental illness, and many women suddenly find themselves thick in the midst of complicated emotions they never believed would accompany becoming a mama. So, important questions to consider are:

1. Do I have a genetic predisposition for depression, anxiety, or mental illness? If the answer is yes, you are at a 50 percent greater risk for developing PPD. Women who have a history of bipolar disorder are at the highest risk of developing postpartum psychosis, the rarest and also most severe postpartum mood disorder. For many women who are struggling, appropriate medication support can be incredibly helpful and important.

2. Are you able to strategize around sleep? Can you get support during the day to nap or at night so that you can get at least four to five hours of uninterrupted sleep each night? Studies have indicated that sleep deprivation may play a greater role in the development of depression and/or anxiety than the temperament of one's baby.
3. Are you getting enough nutrients? It is easy for mom to become depleted during pregnancy, childbirth, and breastfeeding. Adequate nutrition is an important part of your body's ability to make and process necessary "feel good" brain chemicals such as serotonin and dopamine.
4. Are you hydrated? Dehydration and anxiety have been correlated, and many moms, especially breastfeeding moms, are just not hydrating enough.

Social Network: Ours is one of the few societies in which it is assumed (or expected) that mom can and will take care of a babe and everything else on her own. You've heard the saying "It takes a village"? Well, it does! So it's important to seek out the much-needed and deserved support at this time, especially if you have postpartum depression.

1. Can you enlist the aid of friends, family, or hired professionals to help with cooking, cleaning, and even just holding the baby so that you can sleep, shower, or get some time to yourself? Do you know of someone who is willing to set up a "meal train" in which friends and acquaintances drop off much-needed meals several times a week?
2. Do you know other new moms you can talk to during this challenging time? Isolation plagues most new moms, so getting the necessary emotional support is imperative. Research shows that moms groups (therapy support groups or community groups) can decrease symptoms of depression and anxiety in many women.
3. If you are married or partnered, are your relationship needs being met? We know that the first year after having a new baby is often the hardest on relationships, so it is hugely important to tend to these needs. Does your partner need help understanding what you are going through? Is Dad or non-birth Mom suffering from PPD him/herself? Are you able to seek out a trained professional to help navigate some of these relationship challenges?

Psychological Processes: Even if basic needs are being met, the mind can take hold and truly wreak havoc on well-being. Receiving validation, working with a trained therapist, and allowing yourself the care that you need can often help to shift thought patterns that contribute to unwelcome symptoms.

1. Yes, new motherhood is surprisingly difficult for those of us who like to be in control, are perfectionists, or are not expecting the inevitable identity

shifts that come along with becoming a parent. Understanding your triggers around this, being especially kind to yourself, and resetting expectations and priorities so that they are appropriate for this time are imperative.

2. Are past or unresolved issues with your family of origin interfering with your ability to be present with and attach to your own baby? This is an important piece to consider and is usually quite unexpected. The same goes for previous trauma histories, if they exist. Understanding the past's role in the present is hugely important.
3. Are you able to regulate your emotions when necessary? Breathing techniques such as diaphragmatic breathing, progressive relaxation, and guided imagery have been shown to be clinically effective in decreasing depressive and anxiety symptoms.

Of course, of course, of course I *know* none of this is ever as easy as it reads. The support of a trained mental health provider is almost always an important part in a mom's recovery. He or she should be able to help you navigate through these and other important questions as you strive for wholeness again.

When PPD/PPA Treatment Takes Longer Than You'd Like

I know that you want to feel better. Fast! Now! Yesterday! Sooner rather than later. As quickly as possible. That's a given!

For many women, the hardest part of treatment is admitting that you need help. For some, it's picking up the phone and making that first appointment with a therapist. For others, it's taking the plunge and deciding to add medication to your treatment plan. For many, it's the feeling of waiting until things begin to shift and change. This period of waiting (although, truthfully, you are doing so much more than simply "waiting") can feel like decades.

I had a family in my office once who had been struggling for much longer than they would have liked. Mom was ready to have herself back. Dad was ready to have his wife back. The kiddos were ready to have both their mom and dad back. Postpartum depression and anxiety had put their whole family through the ringer.

"Can't we just increase the medication dosage today?" asked Dad. Mom has been taking her meds for five days.

"I just keep waiting to wake up and feel back to normal," says Mom. She has been suffering for quite a long time.

"I know that you both want this all to change so badly," I acknowledge. "So badly that you want a big, red shiny button to push right now that will make everything all better." I know this red, shiny button well. It's like a mirage for the women who come into my office. It sits on the wall to my right, within reach of my chair. I want desperately to push it for every mom I sit with too.

But this simply is not possible. Getting better takes time, hard work, dedication, and strength. Often women who choose to take medication will begin to see a relief in symptoms within about two to three weeks, but for most this is not the finish line. But those moms who follow recommended treatment plans by trained professionals DO GET BETTER! So many moms who come into my office don't believe for a second that they will one day realize that they are in a different place. That they have met their goals of therapy. That they are smiling more, or have more energy, or are more aware of their surroundings. That they do, indeed, have their lives back.

Then the day comes when they look at me with that renewed glow and realize that they do. It's possible. I promise.

VII. FOR FAMILY AND FRIENDS:
How to Support the Mom You Love

If You Think a New Mom Has PPD, Should You Say Something?

Scenario #1: *You are at the playground with your toddler, and you overhear a pregnant mom talking about how sad and anxious she has been feeling. In her conversation with another woman, she mentions that she doesn't know what to do about her increasing sadness.*

Scenario #2: *Your neighbor, whom you do not know extremely well, has just returned from the hospital with her newborn. Like so many brand-new mamas, she looks tired and worn. You ask her how her birth was, and she gets tearful as she talks about her traumatic and unexpected emergency C-section experience that left her baby in the NICU for seven days.*

Scenario #3: *Your childhood friend has a pregnant friend who is in the middle of a divorce and custody battle over her two older children. Your childhood friend, not yet a mother herself, mentions how worried she is about this pregnant mom.*

Scenario #4: *You are at the grocery store, and you overhear two moms talking. One of them is anxiously noting all of the things that worry her about being a mom—the risk of limitless danger that can potentially come to her little one. She mentions choking hazards, air quality, radiation from technology, and pesticides. You overhear her talk about how badly she needs a break but how she trusts no one to help her with her baby. By the end of this short conversation, this mom is sobbing, and no amount of reassurance from her friend seems to help.*

Scenario #5: *A colleague from work has recently told you that she is pregnant. She is overjoyed. She also mentions that she has taken herself off of her medication for a bipolar disorder that she has managed since her late teenage years.*

If confronted with any of these situations, should you step in and share what you know about PPD? Do you share your own experience, even if uninvited?

Whether or not to start a conversation about postpartum mood and anxiety disorders like PPD is such a great dilemma as it speaks to a number of issues that I know recovering and recovered moms contemplate: *Is it okay for me to talk to other moms about postpartum depression and anxiety? How do I talk to others about these issues without assuming that their experience will be exactly like mine? How do I stay away from contributing to fear? What kind of words do I use, and when are the appropriate times to reach out? What if that mom gets angry with me for speaking up about the potential for PPD? What can I do now that will give back to the larger community of women who struggle?*

No textbook answer is available; there is no should or shouldn't about whether or not to initiate a conversation with other moms about what you now know about PPD. But in an attempt to bring some clarity to the confusion around this, I offer the following suggestions and things to consider.

1. How well do you know the mom who is struggling? If you don't know her at all, do you know someone she knows whom you can educate and inform? Sometimes this information is simply best heard from someone a mom trusts, and so seeking out these people can be helpful.
2. What is the setting? A busy playground with many other moms may not be the most appropriate place to approach someone about the risks of PPD. But if you are alone in a park and see someone struggling, it may be that a supportive ear is just what that mama needs in the moment.
3. Being careful about assumption is hugely important. Talking about your experience specifically may be helpful, but it's also useful to speak about women in general and the larger picture of PPD. Using words like "many women" and "moms with newborns" will probably cause less defensiveness than using "you."
4. How far away from your own experience are you? If you are still struggling through your own PPD and are easily triggered, it is best to wait. Sometimes hearing another mom's story about anxiety, scary thoughts, or deep distress can aggravate yours, and protecting your own health is first and foremost.
5. It is important to remember that when someone gets angry at your efforts, it does not necessarily mean she doesn't need, or appreciate, your support and information. In fact, we are often most defensive when we are also most

insecure. If you are worried about another mom's safety or the well-being of her children, it is always okay to attempt to support her and/or reach out to others who may be able to do so. Using respectful and appropriate words is important, as is staying away from assumption. But it is better to reach out and be wrong in a moment of crisis than to step away for fear of making someone angry.

6. Have you done your homework? If you are going to approach someone about PPD, it is important that you know your facts. Giving correct information about the risk factors, warning signs, treatment options, and more is imperative if you are going to attempt to pass along this information at all.
7. Do you have any resources to pass along? While validation and support are super helpful at a time of distress, so is information about where to go for additional support. Knowing ahead of time about a direction to point a mom in is important, whether that is toward online support like Postpartum Progress (postpartumprogress.com) or local support in your area.
8. If and when you do decide to talk to a mom about PPD, it is important you let her know that struggling with postpartum depression is not her fault and that with support she will feel better. Providing hope is imperative.
9. When you make yourself available to moms for this discussion, you may find that you need support for yourself afterward. It can be hard, and often draining, to spend time talking with a mom who is in distress, so making sure that you are able to fill yourself back up afterward is hugely important. Consider having a friend, partner, or therapist to support you around whatever comes up for you in that conversation.

Reaching out to moms who are struggling with PPD is sometimes best done by reaching out to the larger community. If you are a recovered mom who wants to give back and be a support to others, there are limitless ways to do that. Can you write an article for your local newspaper? Contribute a blog post? Give a talk at a local moms group or community center about PPD? Reducing stigma and increasing awareness about postpartum mood and anxiety disorders takes all of us.

Tips for Postpartum Dads, Non-Birth Moms, and Partners

The moms I see in my practice and their partners back home struggle with understandable frustration. In fact, the word "partner" may seem extremely far from the experience of the moms I work with. The first year after having a baby is inevitably challenging for every couple, but add a postpartum mood disorder like postpartum depression, and any resemblance of understanding and communication may seem distant for many couples. It is important to remember that this is usually a case of misunderstanding and lack of information on the part of the non-birth parent. They want to help, and simply don't know how. They want Mom to be happy, and simply don't understand what is happening for her. Giving partners as much information about what is happening to you and your needs at this time is imperative.

Pregnancy and postpartum mood and anxiety disorders affect the whole family. If you are a non-birth parent and partnered with a mom who is struggling, here are some tips that might help you along the way. Remember that you will both get through this with help and support. There is no magic cure, and sometimes recovery seems slow, but things will keep improving if you stick to a plan of health care, support, and communication.

Common Symptoms of Perinatal Depression and Anxiety

- Feeling overwhelmed, exhausted, and insecure
- Crying spells, sadness, hopelessness
- Anger, irritability, frustration
- Repetitive fears and worries

Taking Care of Your Stress and Emotions

- Ask for help, information, and support for yourself. One out of every 10 dads and non-birth mothers will develop symptoms of depression/anxiety in the first year after having a baby.
- Develop a support team for your family. Ask for help. Say YES when they offer.
- Take time for yourself.
- Talk to other families who have come through this.
- Spend time with your baby to develop your own confidence.

How to Help Mom

- Reassure her: This is not her fault; she is not alone; she will get better.
- Encourage her to talk about her feelings, and listen without judgment.
- Help with housework before she asks you.
- Encourage her to take time for herself. Breaks are a necessity; fatigue is a major contributing factor to worsening symptoms.
- Don't expect her to be a super-housewife just because she's home all day.
- Be realistic about what time you'll be home, and come home on time.
- Help her reach out to others for support and treatment.
- Schedule some dates with her and work together to find a babysitter.
- Offer simple affection and physical comfort, but be patient if she is not up for sex. It's normal for her to have a low sex drive with depression, and rest and recovery will help to bring it back.

Dealing with Her Anger and Irritability

- Do what you can to make sure she eats regularly throughout the day because low blood sugar results in a low mood and frustration. Have healthy and easy snacks on hand.
- Do your best to listen for the real request at the heart of her frustration. Reduce conflict by telling her, "I know we can work this out. I am listening."
- Keep the lines of communication open. Verbalize your feelings instead of distancing from her. It is helpful to take a break if your tempers are hot, but do get back to communicating.
- If she is expressing anger in such a way that you can't stay supportive, you might say something like, "I want to listen to you. I know this is important, but I'm having a hard time because you're so mad at me. Can we take a break and talk about it later?"
- Ask her how you can help right now. If she doesn't know, make some suggestions.

VIII. PARENTING:
How to Be Good Enough

How to Be a Good Enough Mother: Why Imperfection Is the Only Way

Perfectionism. Oh, the pressure we put on ourselves to be perfect! Or at least, if not "perfect," then definitely GOOD. The phrase "I feel like such a bad mom" bounces off of the walls in my office every day.

These. Are. Powerful. Words.

But, what do they really mean? What, exactly, is a "good mom" anyway? Is a good mother the one who breastfeeds her baby until he is two years old? Is she the mom who never ever loses her patience? Is this good mom the one who stays home with her kids? Or is she the mom who returns to work and manages to juggle both with grace and ease?

Is a good mom the one who cooks all of her meals from scratch? Is she the mother who always puts others before herself? Is this good mom the one who is constantly smiling and has a perfectly clean house, homemade (organic) cookies on the counter top, and clean, folded laundry put away before anyone notices it was even dirty? Or is she the mom who never feeds her kiddo sugar or lets her watch TV? Is a good mother the one who manages a totally happy marriage that includes frequent sex and date nights and also manages to keep happy and loving siblings from fighting? Is she the one who is always happy, never sad or angry, and definitely not anxious, and who seems to know exactly what to do with her kiddo at every developmental stage? Is she the one whose baby is never crying? Is she the one whose children are always happy, too?

I'd like to meet one of these "good moms." I need her autograph.

While these are extremes, these are also the phrases I have heard many times in the work that I do. This is no joke, people. Most of us carry at least one of these expectations with us into our definitions of "good mom." The catch? Usually these definitions of good motherhood are not ours: They are society's. They come from our own mothers, are the definitions from the books on our bedside table, from our pediatrician, neighbors, partners, or the woman we sat next to at music class.

Donald Winnicott (1896-1971) was a pediatrician and psychoanalyst who, in my opinion, nailed this dilemma on the head. Winnicott studied child development and was a leader in the field of child psychological health. He believed that perfection simply is not perfect. Winnicott spoke and wrote at length about the concept of the "good enough mother": a mother whose mistakes and imperfections lead to the psychological health and important social and emotional development of her children.

From this perspective, mothers actually *need* to be flawed and imperfect so that they can teach their children the importance of repair, so that their children learn not to fear mistakes, and so that they learn the value of repairing—or bringing resolution to—situations or interactions that are flawed. Based on this reasoning, if a mother were always perfect and never made mistakes, she would never give her child the opportunity to learn how to forgive, apologize, learn from mistakes, love unconditionally, and be human. In other words, this child would never learn how to be his or her most true self. Imperfection is good.

So, with that definition, I have a project for you:

Hear, hear!!!

1. On a piece of paper, write down everything that comes to mind when you think about your own definition of what it means to be a "good enough mother." I encourage you to be mindful of what comes at you. Are the pieces that go into your definition yours, or are they someone else's? For this exercise, give yourself permission to own this definition, regardless of what others might say or think. What do *you* believe goes into being a good enough mom? Please, please, please avoid words such as *always* and *never.*
2. Go through your list and ask yourself if you are doing or being anything on your list. Try your best to think of at least one thing or one time that you have met each piece of your definition. For example, if "being loving" is on your list, what exactly does that look like and how have you "been loving" to your baby?

3. Place your list next to your bed. Each night, ask yourself if you have engaged in any of the "good enough mom" elements that you have noted. My guess is that you have.

In fact, I can bet most of what I own on the fact that each one of you reading this is a darn good enough mom. You just might not have been noticing.

Eight Ways to Be a Good Mother Instead of a Perfect One

I think it's fair to say that each one of us enters motherhood with a set of beliefs or expectations about what it means to be a good mother. We develop these beliefs from the pressure of our communities and society as a whole, the experiences with our own parents, and the expectations of friends, family, and media. These outside influences can have so much power and sway over us that when we finally do become mothers ourselves, it is unbearably difficult to listen to our own ideas of what this "good mom" thing is all about. So difficult, in fact, that anxiety, depression, and overwhelming emotion can latch on like crazy to our new identity.

I want to share a brief story with you about a mom I saw in my office once. This mom has given me permission to share her process around the topic of being a good mother, because it gives such a clear example of the ways in which perfectionist thinking and unachievable expectations can lead to distress.

Dana (not her real name) came to my office when her baby was about four months old. She was attractive, articulate, and also very scared by the unpleasant thoughts and anxieties she had been feeling since her baby was born. Dana described sleepless nights of worry, her lack of appetite, fear and insecurity about being alone with her baby, and the pure distress that was accompanying her early motherhood. She told me, through tears and obvious guilt, that she was having very scary thoughts of hurting her baby or herself—thoughts that terrified her, she said, because she did not want her baby or herself to be hurt. Dana felt that her thoughts and emotions were out of control and that she was going "crazy." She described a traumatic delivery in which an emergency C-section led her to believe that she would not make it through alive. "I realized that I needed to be willing to give up my life for my baby," she said.

When Dana's symptoms were being managed through a combination of medication and therapy support, we began the process of identifying beliefs about motherhood that might be adding to her distress. I have an exercise that I do with moms in my office that asks them to write down all the things they believe go into being a "good enough" mom. Dana's first list looked like this:

1. A "good enough" mom:
2. Loves her child unconditionally
3. Never hurts her child
4. Always does what is best for her child
5. Always puts her child's needs before her own
6. Always wants to be around her child

7. Should always feel that the most important thing in the world is her child
8. Should always be willing to give up anything for her child
9. Should be happy staying home with her kids all day
10. Never resents her child
11. Should feel the only thing she needs in her life to feel happy is her child
12. Should completely define herself as a person through motherhood
13. Shouldn't feel bored spending time with her child
14. Should feel happy and overjoyed every time she looks at her child
15. Should never think about how enjoyable her life was before kids
16. Should be able to handle kids all day without needing breaks (luxury)
17. Shouldn't feel unhappy at night when up with her child

As I said to Dana at the time, this list makes me anxious when I read it, and so I can only imagine what it must have felt like to her to believe that all of these things were a necessary part of mothering.

The *shoulds*

The *shouldn'ts*

The *always*

They make it hard to breathe.

Helping her realize this did not take long, and Dana was quick to acknowledge that as she wrote down these beliefs about motherhood, these expectations looked too high. When I asked her where she learned them, she said she always believed that this is how her mom felt and what her mom believed when she was growing up. Do you know what her mom said when Dana showed her this "good mother" list? "Oh my ... no mother feels this way!"

We worked through this. It was not easy for Dana to come up with a more realistic, comfortable, and fair list of what it means to be a "good enough" mom, but once she was able to really examine what she believes, she came up with this:

A good mother, often called a "good enough" mom, *does her best to:*

1. Teach her child how to live life to the fullest
2. Be available for her children when they need her
3. Teach her child the importance of self-worth
4. Provide food, shelter, and love
5. Be a good example to her children

6. Make time to have fun with her kids
7. Allow room for her children to make mistakes and learn from them
8. Teach her children how to love unconditionally
9. Pretty big difference, right?
10. No shoulds, shouldn'ts, always, or nevers.
11. No perfection.

Dana got to a place where she was doing much better. Her panic attacks and scary thoughts decreased. She was better able to access feelings of hope and optimism, and she enjoyed her baby more. Her medication helped with the biochemical imbalances that added to her symptoms of postpartum anxiety and OCD, and her more realistic idea of what it means to be a good mother to her kiddo took some of the pressure off.

We all do this. Each of us enters motherhood with some idea of what we "should" do in this new and often overwhelming role. While many of those things may be entirely appropriate, many others may be entirely unachievable.

I encourage you to ask yourself what it is that you believe goes into being a "good enough" mom to your kiddo and write down your own list. Take note of the "shoulds" and the "always'" and whether or not you are listing ideas that are truly yours or whether they are someone else's (breastfeeding your baby versus providing nutritious food whenever possible might be a good example), or your assumptions of someone else's.

My guess is that when you truly examine your beliefs about motherhood, you'll discover a path that frees you to be exactly the kind of mother your child needs.

The Hardest Part of Parenting

It's not all of the annoying logistics—the nonstop breast- and bottle-feeding, the dirty diapers, the laundry, the constant cleaning up of messes.

It's not the high-pitched crying and whining and constant, never-ending needing of something.

It's not the crazy-making around how to discipline and teach and mentor and try as best we can to raise somewhat kind and functioning little people.

It's not even the fact that we have to somehow keep them alive. Or the reality of lost alone time.

The hardest thing about parenting is this: It is not our job to prevent our children from feeling pain. Our job is, actually, to allow for their pain and to walk them through it.

I might be just speaking for myself, but I don't think so. In all of the years of work that I have done supporting mothers, in all of my personal relationships with other mothers in my life, and as a mother myself, I'm pretty sure that this one is the hardest.

It is not our job to prevent our kids from feeling pain.

We must make space for our kids to feel the pain that comes with being human.

Our children will feel pain throughout their lives. They will experience pain and grief and loss and sadness and anger and worry and uncertainty, and we are not meant to protect them from that. Far from it. It is actually our job to allow their pain to exist and to walk with them through it to the other side. You know why? Because it is our job to teach them what it means to be human, and humans feel pain. Often.

Ugh.

Somehow, we have lost respect for this part of being human. **We want our kids to be brave and resilient and curious and strong, and yet we seem to think that by spending our time trying to prevent them from experiencing pain, we are helping them get to these places.** Of course, this isn't the way it works. Bravery and resiliency and curiosity and strength can only be born out of grief and loss and pain and hardship. **Without the pain, there is simply no practice in resiliency.**

Our kiddo comes home from school and is tearful because her buddy wouldn't sit with her at lunch. His friend didn't invite him to his birthday party. Her pet dies. We can't be available for his school play because of a work meeting. She doesn't make the sports team. He forgets to study for a test and fails. She witnesses an argument between you and her other parent, and she worries you will split up. You do split up, and he now has parents who are divorced.

And we so often think, *Shit, it is my one job to prevent my kiddo from experiencing pain, and I couldn't even do that.*

So, we call the parents. We reach out to the teacher. We contact the coach. We overcompensate because of the missed play and our guilt around it. We hide our distress around our own sadness. We do whatever we possibly can to step in and cushion those little people whom we love so much from feeling any of it.

But this, my friends, is a disservice.

Instead, it is our job to give them a place to cry, to be angry, and to feel uncertain. It is our job to validate and hold their hand and give them hugs and remind them that we know they are okay even when they feel so awful. It is our job to make room for their own problem-solving (with our help when they want it, of course). We have to bite our tongues and refrain from fixing it all for them. We have to just be in the pain with them. Then we must celebrate their resilience when they find their way through.

Call me crazy, but *this* is the part of parenting that feels the hardest. Because each time our hearts break just a little bit with theirs. So we too need to rely on our resiliency and bravery and curiosity and strength to get through. To show them that it's possible.

When the Crying Just Doesn't Stop

As if the first few days, weeks, and months of caring for a new baby weren't challenging enough! We all know how it goes: Your baby cries and cries, and no matter what you try, you can't seem to find the magic button to soothe, calm, and quiet that little bundle. You count the minutes. The hours. The days. The weeks. When, oh when, will that magic three-month mark hit? You go through the list: Is she wet? You change her. Is he hungry? You feed him. Does she have gas? You burp her. Is it the dairy, wheat, or soy? You alter your diet. Is he uncomfortable? You move him around. Is she sick? You take her to the pediatrician. Is he too hot? Too cold? Is her onesie itching her? Does he need to be bounced? Held in the football position? Should you take her outside? No, wait, should you take her back in? You try everything you can think of. Your legs hurt from doing squats, and your arms hurt from carrying her. Soon, you lose faith, and you probably begin to wonder if it is you. You ask yourself all kinds of questions: *Why can't I give my baby what she needs? Am I a bad mother? Why is this easier for everyone else? What is wrong with me?*

Soon, you may even be regretting your choice to have kids. Or considering leaving your partner. Or thinking frequently about just running away.

We know that fussy babies cause the greatest risk for *shaken baby syndrome* and infant death. Now, of course not every parent with a fussy or colicky baby gets to this point, but it is common for any parent who is in this situation to understand how that could happen to someone who wasn't in control of his or her actions and impulses. The bottom line is that caring for a baby who cries and cries for no apparent reason can be overwhelmingly intense for anyone. When you add sleep deprivation and shifting hormones on top of this already stressful situation, having a colicky baby can be downright debilitating.

So... find help. Erikson Institute's The Fussy Baby Network is fabulous. They offer a "warm" line (888-431-BABY) that takes calls from around the world. They also offer in-home visits for families in the Chicago Metropolitan Area. As with any challenge of new motherhood/parenthood, please don't wait to get the support you need. Being a new mama is hard enough. (See resources at the end of this book.)

By the way, just as a reminder: Being overwhelmed and frustrated by a new baby with colic is certainly no reflection of your love for that new baby. We can all love our children and not necessarily love every aspect of parenting. Please allow yourself to get the support that you need knowing, while you do so, that needing this support says nothing about the kind of mother you are. Except, of course, that you care enough to get the help you and your family deserve.

The Working Mom's Dilemma

Like people, attitudes around returning to work (or not) after a baby is born come in all shapes and sizes. For some, returning to work is about as unimaginable as the sky falling, and the mere thought of the realistic need to do so brings with it a shed of tears and heartache. For others, returning to work brings great relief, as it offers a break from the stresses and isolation of being home and provides a chance to reconnect with an old self. Some women have no other option but to return to work and are saddened by the fact that they aren't able to choose to be home with their little one. Others make the choice to stay home, but are then faced with the new identity shifts that come with their role as a stay-at-home mom. Some women feel great pressure to get back into the working field. Others feel great pressure to stay home. Some women feel guilty for their desire to stop working. Others feel guilty for their desire to be away from their baby. The situations are as numerous as the moms. One pretty universal experience exists, however: Nearly every mom is affected by this "choice" as most of us find ourselves smack in the middle of a dilemma that comes along with being a woman with a baby in today's working world.

So, how does an overtired, vulnerable, perhaps postpartum depressed or anxious mom manage the string of emotions that come with this dilemma? How, on Earth, does a mom who must-return-to-work-but-doesn't-feel-ready do it?

Not easily, I am afraid.

I'm not sure that we consider the realities of this challenge when we are excitedly anticipating the arrival of a new baby. One of the most common shifts that a woman goes through once she becomes a mother is the shift in her identity. The once expected "oh, I'll just return to work and jump back into where I left off" doesn't quite match up. Not only is it simply not that easy emotionally, but many women also "feel" different—different, perhaps, than they were when they packed up their stuff and headed out the door toward maternity leave or put their career path on hold. The toughest part may be that all the people who were left back at work won't necessarily understand this. While this identity shift may not be drastic, it is certainly unsettling for many women, and negotiating this transition can lead to anxiety and depression for some.

Many moms, approximately 20%, will suffer from postpartum depression or anxiety in the first year after having a baby, and this often makes returning to work feel even more complex. Hopefully these women have sought out treatment and support, have a resemblance of grounding again, and are able to make this decision confidently. Others, unfortunately, suffer alone and are plagued by an extra layer of anxiety around this transition. On top of all that, one of the symptoms for many women with PPD is a difficulty in making decisions, so you can imagine how stressful this reality must be.

Following are a few strategies that may help lead to a relatively "smooth" transition, whether this transition is toward or away from work. These come with the disclaimer that "relatively" is the word of choice here. Transitions are, by definition, bumpy. Most moms who must make a decision around whether or not to return to work feel ungrounded for a while—whether this work takes them away from their babies or finds them right in the middle of Baby-Land.

1. **Even if you think you are excited about returning to work, take time off—as much time as your job will allow and as much time as you can afford.** Every woman needs to give herself time to settle in after becoming a mother. Rushing back to work too soon is often the breaking point for many women who assume that they must "have it all together" more quickly than is reasonably possible.
2. **If you are able to afford help when you are home, do it.** The shift from working at work to working at home can leave many moms exhausted and emotionally torn. Many moms forget that taking time for self-care serves not only themselves but also their babies and families. So, if a co-parent isn't able to lend a hand, or if you are a single mom, find a friend, neighbor, family member, or sitter to be home with your baby while you get in a nap, a bit of exercise, time with your friends, a date night, a massage, or whatever else fills you up.
3. If it would be useful to you, **ask your childcare provider to keep a log of your baby's activities, including sleeping, eating, and pooping time, temperament, and activity.** This will help you feel a bit more in the loop when you return after a day away. Being able to have an image of your baby when you are not with him or her can be hugely comforting.
4. **If you work close to home, consider a lunch-break visit.** But consider this cautiously. Many moms find that a break in the day to hold, soothe, or feed a baby makes the time away more manageable. But many also find that this visit only makes things tough again when it is time to go. So give it a try, but be kind to yourself if this makes you feel worse, rather than better.
5. **Find partners at work.** It can be incredibly validating to connect with other women who are in your shoes. Whether this is someone whose children are now grown or who has a baby right alongside of you, building your strength through the support of others is invaluable.
6. **Remember that everything is hard in the beginning.** It will get easier. I had a mom in my private practice who cried frequently about her need to return to work from the moment her son was born. She spent six weeks mourning the day that she would leave him with someone other than herself. Then, guess what? She found that after the first day or two, she actually liked her

time away. Within a couple of weeks, she talked happily about the relative ease she was experiencing. She found that being with a crying baby when she was home was much easier when she had a break away for a while.

7. 7. **Think outside of the box.** Sometimes this requires an extra person to help get creative, but so often we get stuck in the "either-or" trap without realizing that we have many options. Some moms are able to take a fifth day off by fulfilling their work requirements in four long days. Others find that they are actually able to work from home part of the time. Some decide that decreasing their hours permanently and being at work part-time is an option. Some make the decision to find a different job altogether that offers flex hours and allows them to work at home.
8. **If you suffer from PPD, continue to get support.** This is so important. This goes right along with #2 and self-care. It is easy to feel like "there is no longer time" for therapy, moms groups, or whatever else you have been doing to get well, but please don't go down this dead-end path. If you are a PPD sufferer, you need your support and treatment more than ever through this transition.
9. **Embrace what feels like it works best for you, with as little guilt as possible.** Babies need present-minded and happy moms, so if this means that you feel better when you have time away at work, then shed the guilt about being away from your baby. If you have always been career driven, and now want and are financially able to embrace an opportunity to be a full-time mom (yes, I know, even working moms are full-time moms), then toss out your work attire with confidence. Sometimes this is easier said than done, so recruit the help of your partner, a friend, or a therapist.
10. **Remember that decades of research have shown us that what babies need most from a parent is empathetic attunement—even more than physical presence.** So, in other words, it is not the quantity of time with your baby that makes the difference, but the quality. You can still give your baby everything he or she needs even if you aren't with your baby 24-7.

Be sure to check out the Resources section to find additional support.

Yoga, Parenting, Life, and Taking Ourselves a Bit Less Seriously

When my daughters were small, Sunday mornings were my mornings "off." They were my mornings to have some space, to take my time getting from here to there, to remember what it feels like to be a woman and not just a mother or wife or perinatal mental health expert, and to be as present as possible while also taking some time to look back at the week past and forward at the one to come. Let me be clear: *I love my family. And my work.* With every part of my being. But without those Sunday mornings off and the time to take for me, I became instantly overloaded.

One Sunday I rode my bike to yoga, as I did every week that I could, to the class and the teacher that I looked forward to when my week started each Monday. It was a crisp but sunny morning in Boulder. A lovely one.

But as soon as I walked into the yoga studio that I knew so well, I became immediately grumpy. My regular teacher was away, and there was a new one standing in whom I did not know nor, truthfully, care to know that Sunday morning. Not only was the teacher new, but he was shuffling us into a circular formation for practice rather than the standard front-facing rows, which meant that I was not able to claim my usual spot (yes, I too get that "creature of habit" thing). So, to summarize, I went instantaneously from cheerful to heavyhearted, just like that.

I swear, this teacher was reading my mind. He began the class talking about change and transition and the discomfort that it puts us in (um, yeah). He invited us on that Sunday morning to be open to what *is* rather than to be discouraged by what *isn't*. To tell you the truth, I may have rolled my eyes a bit. *But this is my yoga!* I thought to myself.

So, he began class. Sun salutations. Yoga and breath flow. He made some jokes. He laughed a bit. He pushed us harder than I expected and then also reminded us to listen to our own bodies and not compare ourselves to those on their mats around us.

Then, Dear Readers, the most eye-opening thing happened. He told us to sigh. Loudly. He told us to exhale a big, loud, "Oh Man!" as we moved ourselves back into downward dog. Understandably on this early Sunday morning, very few people obliged. My guess is that there were other eye rolls and probably lots of grumpy self-talk. But then he said, "Okay class, if sighing loudly and saying 'Oh Man' in yoga is living on the edge, then I encourage you to ask yourself why."

So, I did. Why was it that I was letting my morning be ruined by my own expectations and judgments and opinions? Why was I giving this yoga teacher and this circular formation so much bloody power over my cheerfulness? Why was sighing and yelling "Oh Man" taking on the extreme level of living on the edge? Well, because I was letting it.

And so you know what I did? I sighed. I exclaimed a big, colorful "Oh Man!" With that, my morning turned around.

Why am I taking the time to share this little Sunday morning yoga story with you? Because I realized that it is so very easy to begin to take myself and life around me more seriously than I need to. This is (as always) so much easier said than done if you are really struggling with more than a yoga class—if you are suffering and feeling hopeless and discouraged. But friends, we all allow ourselves to interfere with our own potential from time to time. Can we giggle more? Can we make fun of ourselves when appropriate? Can we catch ourselves letting expectation ruin what *is* by putting unnecessary attention onto what *isn't*? Can we skip down the sidewalk when we are alone just for the silliness of it? Can we let go of the need to have things just so and, instead, let out a loud, rambunctious "Oh yeah!"?

It's worth a try.

Three Steps That Turn Your Mistakes in Motherhood into Wins

Let's start with the facts: If you are like me and most other women, you make a million mistakes as a mom.

I actually don't think I am exaggerating. These mistakes happen whether you are a brand-new mom or a very seasoned one. Of course these mistakes happen across the board for dads, too. **So many of us enter motherhood (parenthood!) thinking that we need to be perfect. Like, if we aren't, if we mess up somehow, we will mess up our kids.** These mistakes come in all shapes and sizes. Big or small. As big as screaming at our kid in a moment of rage and uncertainty to, God forbid, checking our email while our baby is playing next to us on the floor.

We worry that we are the worst mothers in the world. We worry that we are scarring our children for life. We think all other parents on the planet have some recipe to "perfect parenting" that we cannot, for the life of us, find.

Okay. I'm here to save the day.

Actually, science is here to save the day. I'm just the messenger.

Pediatrician and psychoanalyst Donald Winnicott, psychiatrist Daniel Siegel, researcher and professor Brené Brown, and many others have spent their careers studying the ways that parents and children interact. They have studied what matters most in "good parenting" and what, actually, has the potential to cause damage that will impact children's mental health moving forward. Their research and data are consistent and clear:

Perfect parenting can cause harm.

Making mistakes in parenting can build strong attachments and a strong sense of self for your child as he or she grows up.

I mean, phew, right?

So, what does this mean? **It means that the "perfect" mom who is always a step ahead, who makes sure her child is never uncomfortable—never hungry, sad, disappointed, or unsure—sends a message to her child that he is not okay, that he needs her all the time, and that relationships are built on perfection and success, and that imperfection in relationships is a sign that something is terribly wrong. It means that the mom who makes mistakes is sending the message that mistakes are part of being human—we all make them all the time. When we suggest to our children that mistakes are bad, we set them up for a lot of suffering (and dare I say therapy) later on. And guess what? What we say to our kids doesn't really matter at all, if what we are doing is something different.** We can tell our four-year-old that spilling her milk is okay, but if she comes into the kitchen later and sees us swearing under our breath for spilling something ourselves, then that is what she will learn.

Making. Mistakes. Is. Important.

So, what does this look like in real time? How can we use our mistakes to help our children and our relationships with them become stronger?

Learn to forgive yourself for the mistakes you make, big or small. Remind yourself that you are human. Take a deep breath. Try an "oops" or "yikes," rather than a "I'm so stupid" or "What is wrong with me?"

Repair. When you make a mistake with your kiddo (yell, miss it when he needs something from you, get to school pickup late, emotionally retreat at a time when you are preoccupied by your own stuff), own it. Say that you are sorry. Let them know that it makes sense that they are angry, disappointed, or sad. Remind them that you will do your part in making sure it doesn't happen again or on a regular basis. (Then, do your work to follow through on this.)

When your kiddo makes a mistake, take a deep breath before reacting. Remind her that all humans make mistakes. Take a moment or two to get down at her level, look her in the eyes, and tell her that it is okay. After that moment you can get her help in cleaning up the spill and make a plan to avoid the same mistake in the future. But first, give her permission to be imperfect.

What this offers our children is the freedom to be real, full-blown, imperfect humans. Children who are given permission to make mistakes actually grow up making fewer stupid ones. Truly. This is because they learn from their mistakes rather than developing a sense of shame. This also reminds our kids that they can trust us to love them unconditionally—that our love is not dependent on their performance. And this contributes to their ability to love themselves unconditionally, which is a major key in mental health. Finally, this mistake and repair experience helps our children to be fully seen by us, which is incredibly important in healthy bonding and attachment.

So, there you have it. Take a deep breath. Forgive yourself. Be human. And help your child grow into that person you hope they will be. Mistakes and all.

Healthy Moms Have Healthy Boundaries

We are all told we need healthy boundaries, but how many of us really have them? And what is a boundary anyway?

These questions are pretty much everywhere right now. Our country has emerged from a pandemic in which work/life/family/self, have all kind of blurred into one big ball of chaos. During the pandemic, our typical self-care practices went out the window with the closing of yoga and fitness studios, gyms, nail salons, restaurants, movie theaters, massage studios, community centers, day care, and school, and suddenly we found ourselves, well, boundary-less. It's not a good feeling. It's not good for our mental health.

We need to refocus on creating the kind of boundaries that allow us to sustain mental and physical health. It's a good time to do it. So many of us are asking ourselves who we want to be as we come back out into a world that has proven itself to be unpredictable and risky. We are ready to be healthy. We are ready to be brave.

But where to start? Are you struggling with wondering what a boundary is? Welcome to the party.

Let's muddle through this together.

Here is what a boundary is not:

A boundary is not a barrier. A boundary is not meant as a way to separate yourself from others. A boundary is not a punishment or a way of getting back at someone you are hurt by or angry with. A boundary is not a withholding of self. A boundary is not selfish.

Here is what a boundary is:

A boundary is a proactive way to show up as your most true and authentic self. A boundary is in service of the whole community. A boundary is an act of generosity as it helps to protect others from the part of yourself that is destructive and reactive. A boundary is a way to create the space that you need to be healthy and well. A boundary is self-full in a way that supports you to have what you need to give back to the world your greatest, most creative, most generous self.

But here is what I want to yell from the treetops. **As human beings, it is our responsibility to learn what we each need to be mentally and physically well. Once we know what those things are, it is our job to ask for what we need.** It is our job to say "no" to the things that get in the way of that health and wellness. It is our job to advocate for ourselves. It is *not* our job to manage the thoughts and feelings of others when it comes to these needs, requests, and boundaries. It is *not* our job to convince others that our boundaries make sense and are justified. It is *not* our job to make sure that others accept the boundaries that we set. These efforts are destined to fail anyway.

Three Choices

IT'S A PARENTING TOOL.

Your kiddo is being a pain in the butt. I'm sure you have all been there. She is yelling at her brother. He is throwing a tantrum because you forgot to wash his favorite T-shirt. Mean words and flying appendages are everywhere, and your head is about to explode.

"You have three choices," you say. *"1. Be kind, 2. Be polite, or 3. Take some space."*

Three choices. None of them involve causing harm to one's self or someone else. Choice #1 involves leaning in, engaging, asking questions. Choice #2 involves being somewhat neutral but also respectful—a quiet presence. Then choice #3 involves honoring a capacity (or lack thereof) for connection in the moment, and if the ability to stay kind or polite isn't available, the option to take space is always available. This choice involves walking away.

"Three choices. Which do you choose, kiddo?"

If you stay consistent with this, it works. Seriously. Try it.

But what if we used this for ourselves as well? What if we told ourselves in moments of stress, frustration, irritability, disappointment, and anger that we had three choices?

I can be kind... I can be polite... or I can take some space!

What if the choice to take space—to walk away—was in service to everybody involved? What if that choice was totally okay? What if that choice was considerate and generous and caring toward both yourself and the other person?

What if being mean, aggressive, violent, and shaming toward yourself and others was never one of the choices?

Would it help?

Three choices. Which do you choose?

Intentional Parenting: Apology and Ownership

Many of us were not taught the importance of owning our mistakes in life, especially with our children. Many of us were not raised by parents who owned their own mistakes, and many of our parents may never have apologized for anything. We might have been led to believe that we should not admit to failure and uncertainty when we are parenting. We think that our children's respect comes from a sense that we know everything, are right all the time, and are never vulnerable.

Let me burst that false bubble as quickly as I can.

In all relationships, including parenting, ownership for wrongdoing and taking responsibility for our choices goes a long, long way in building trust, respect, and strong attachment. We model this important trait to our children all the time. Through our own actions, we teach them the value of reflection and empathy and responsibility. Or, we teach them the value of self-preservation and perfection and power over another.

Which do you choose?

But not all apologies are created equal:

"I'm sorry but (you made me do it, or you deserved it, or I was angry, or [fill in the blank])" is very defensive.

"I'm sorry that you feel like I (didn't listen, or disappointed you, or [fill in the blank])" is very blaming.

"I'm sorry that you (are feeling so sensitive, or can't handle criticism, or don't know how to take a joke)" is very dismissive.

Just: ***"I'm sorry."***

"I'm sorry that I lost my patience." I'm sorry that I hurt your feelings." "I'm sorry that I wasn't paying attention." "I'm sorry that I spoke to you that way."

Just "I'm sorry."

What is the most perfect response to an apology, whether it is you or your child who is receiving the apology?

You've got it: ***"Thank you."***

Not *"It's okay,"* or *"Don't worry about it,"* or *"It's not a big deal."* Just: ***"Thank you."***

Then everyone can move on, knowing that humans aren't perfect and that when we can own our part in conflict and repair, we are left that much stronger and worthy of respect.

But don't take my word for it, of course. Give it a try. See what happens.

Intentional Parenting: Reflection

If you are reading this then you are already on the right track.

If you are curious about what it means to parent intentionally, then you likely already are. There is a difference between *"being a parent"* and *"parenting,"* and if you have gotten this far, then you can pat yourself on the back because not all parents are curious enough to read books like this. You, however, are *"parenting."* You, my friend, are definitely in the "intentional parent" community.

But we don't always know what that means. **By definition, being intentional means that we are being deliberate in our actions—that we are doing the things we do on purpose, for a reason, and with awareness.** From where I sit in my office, parenting unintentionally—without awareness and without purpose—has pretty big consequences. We feel pretty bad about ourselves. We feel lost and annoyed and overwhelmed. We often react without thinking. Our kids suffer. The reality is that every single one of us has been there.

Most of us want to be *good enough* parents.

One important concept in "good enough parenting" that will lead both you and your child(ren) toward solid, secure, and healthy growth and relationships is this:

REFLECTION

Reflective parenting, which uses curiosity, self-awareness, and self-compassion, allows a parent to see the world both through his or her perspective as well as his or her kiddo's perspective.

If you are a reflective parent, you ask yourself, *"How is what I am doing and saying right now impacting my kid? How might my kid be interpreting what I am saying and doing?"* As a reflective parent, you understand that your child's behavior (and your own!) is a reflection of how your child (and you) feels. You value emotions and feelings as a part of being human. You understand that the choices you make as a human and a parent fundamentally impact your child's sense of self and the world. You understand that no human (including you!) is perfect, that people make mistakes, and that when we pay attention, we can learn and grow from those mistakes. As a reflective parent, you, well, *reflect* on how you are parenting your child and what your child's experiences might be with you as their mom or dad. You are inquisitive and curious, but you also understand that the goal is not necessarily to know the answers, but to wonder.

Does that sound like a lot of work?

It's actually a lot less work than suffering through confusion and feeling bad about yourself and your kid. Trust me. I've done the experiment. Many times.

Here is what you need to do to engage in reflective parenting:

Pause. As a reflective parent, you must be willing to slow down and pay attention.

Observe. Watch and notice with compassion what is happening for both you and your child.

Be curious. Think *what, why*, and *how.*

What might my child be feeling right now?

Why might he/she be feeling that way and responding that way?

How are my words and actions impacting my child?

Those of us who weren't raised this way will have a harder time parenting this way. It can feel foreign and unnatural and very, very slow. But it pays off. And, to be clear, reflective parents definitely set boundaries and hold their kids accountable for their behavior. Reflective parenting is not a form of discipline. It is a form of relating to another human whom you care about and want to be in a strong and healthy relationship with.

On Motherhood...and Supermom

Mother's Day was coming to a close. My husband was in California for work, and I spent my second Mother's Day in a row alone with my two spectacular daughters. I can't tell a lie: I spent much of the earlier part of the day simply feeling sorry for myself—no breakfast in bed, no mom's day off yoga class, no sweet reminders from my husband about how appreciated I am. Truthfully, feeling sorry for myself is probably an understatement. I was kind of pissed.

Then, thanks to all of the wonderful women I work with each week, I was reminded that I needed to practice what I preach in my office. The more I thought about how disappointed I was that I wasn't being publicly celebrated in my pajamas, the more down I felt. All that I really wanted was to feel great on Mother's Day. So I looked at the two faces on the other side of the breakfast table and took charge. I decided that on that day *I* was going to celebrate myself.

And all of you.

You see, motherhood drives me. Not just the day in and day out of the joys and frustrations of raising my two young daughters, but that huge, all-consuming FACT of motherhood. I have made the choice to be one myself. I have molded my career after working with moms. I think and talk about motherhood all day every day whether it is with myself, the women with whom I work, my colleagues, or my dearest friends. It is literally what I feel most passionate about in the whole wide world.

Human life on Earth would not exist without mothers. No world population. Not. One. Person. Would. Exist. Without. Mothers.

I mean, whoa. We are important!!!

The term "mother" is all encompassing, isn't it? On that particular Mother's Day, I asked moms to share their views on the definition of "mother," and I received one response that I will share here:

I am my children's everything. I am a Supermom even when I don't feel like it or look like it.

I have thought about this response so many times as Mother's Day hits each year and I celebrate myself and the mothers of the world.

She is her children's everything: Without her, her children would be lost. Her responsibility to them as growing little people who will become adults perhaps with children of their own is overwhelming at times. Her children depend on her for security, consistency, trust, love, and guidance. Their health depends on her health. Therefore, her health is of the highest importance. *She is her children's everything.* So she needs to be as well as she is able. Healthy. Happy. Fulfilled. Full. She needs to be happy and healthy and well to the best of her ability for herself whether she works inside or outside of the home. So that she has the immense amounts of energy that it takes to give to the little people who depend on her.

Women who do not feel this way deserve to get the support they need to feel better. This is not to say, of course, that moms need to feel great all the time. That simply would not be human. But if moms truly are their kids' everything, they need her. They need her to be her best self. So does she.

She is a Supermom even if she doesn't feel like it or look like it. I love this part. I have written about Supermom before, although I have written about her from the position of "she doesn't exist." I think I like this perspective even better. What this mom was saying is that **we are all Supermoms.**

Each one of us who is a mom is a Supermom when we are feeling our best. When we are not. We are Supermoms when we are dressed up for work or date night and also when we haven't showered for several days, slept for several days, or cooked for several days. We are Supermoms when we are patient and also when we have lost our tempers. We are Supermoms when we are making our children's Halloween costumes or baking our kiddo's birthday cake from scratch and also when we are banking on store-bought everything. We are Supermoms when we make it to the gym or run a marathon and also when the word exercise is hidden away with our pre-kid wardrobes. We are Supermoms when we are working all day at the office and also when we are home all day with our kids. We are Supermoms when we breastfeed our children through toddlerhood and also when we formula-feed from the start. We are Supermoms when we deliver babies naturally and also when we have assisted births or C-sections. We are Supermoms when we have mastered a clean house and folded laundry and also when the dishes are piled high and our children are in the same filthy outfit for the third day in a row. We are Supermoms when we finish a novel or the *Sunday Times* and also when we have forgotten how to read or have eyes only for books whose font fills half a page. We are Supermoms when we are discussing politics or the environment and also when talking about nothing other than poop. We are Supermoms when we are emotionally well and also when we are not. We are Supermoms when we have avoided or are over our debilitating bouts of postpartum depression and also when we are right smack in the middle of it.

We are *all* Supermoms!

Move over blue bikini with the stars.

So as you read this, I salute all of you Supermoms out there. We make the world go 'round, sisters. Whether you are riding the wave or being swallowed up by the white water, we are all part of the same team and need to look out for each other. Every second of every day. We need to watch out for ourselves and we need to watch out for our neighbors because Batman and Robin are nothing compared to us.

The world needs us to be well.

Whether today is officially Mother's Day or not, Happy Mother's Day. I am honored to be one of you.

IX: WHEN YOU ARE AT THE END OF YOUR ROPE:

Know That You Are Not Alone

To the Postpartum Depression Moms Suffering in Silence

Too often, I have moms calling my office in desperate need of postpartum depression support 10 or 12 months after giving birth to their little ones. These are not the moms who felt good for the first seven or eight months only to be hit full force with symptoms of postpartum depression or anxiety upon weaning or when menstruating for the first time since having their baby. These are the moms who have been struggling on and off for months and who have waited until a breaking point to reach out. What all these moms tell me is this: *"I am so ashamed to be needing help like this, but I just can't take it anymore."*

These are the moms who, to the outside world, seem to be doing just fine. They pull themselves out of bed in the morning, have their showers, and pull on a clean set of clothes in order to impress others in their lives. Inside, though, they feel like complete impostors. They feel good enough to hold conversations, smile at the checkout clerk, and return emails, but find themselves in the fetal position when no one is looking. These are the moms who feel terrible for several days and then feel better the next, so they tell themselves that they must be fine until they are hit, again, by several days of near intolerable suffering (once again, behind closed doors). These are the moms who are afraid to let their partners know the depths of their despair for fear of judgment by the people who are supposed to know them the best.

Yes. I worry about these moms. A lot.

What we know is that women who struggle postpartum anywhere along the spectrum from very mild postpartum adjustment to very severe postpartum psychosis, who reach out for support from an appropriately trained mental health provider, and who follow treatment recommendations do get well. Thankfully, many of the moms who are in severe crises will get help sooner rather than later because friends, family members, or their health providers will be able to tell from the outside that something is drastically wrong. So, while I don't at all like the fact that women who fall into the more extreme end of the spectrum suffer, I do know that the impetus for reaching out is often shared by others around them because it is impossible to hide their suffering. The responsibility does not lie solely on them.

Then there are the women on the other far end of the spectrum—those who feel ill-at-ease in their new roles, whose biochemistry is off enough to increase their feelings of vulnerability but resilient enough to balance itself out on its own over a fairly short period of time. I don't worry so much about these moms with mild symptoms either because they are usually the moms who will find a community, pick up mom-baby yoga, or openly discuss their challenges with others.

It's the moms in the middle—the ones who seem to get lost in the crowd of postpartum women. These moms have me in a real fluster.

It's not that I can't help them to recover, because I can. Those of us who work in the field of perinatal mood and anxiety disorders like postpartum depression know what to do to help these postpartum depression moms feel better. We know what questions to ask in taking a full history and inventory of symptoms, risk factors, and internal and external conflicts that may be interfering with their ability to feel the way they want to. We know how to partner with these moms and how to advise them toward recovery.

But what we can't do is take away the months of suffering that took place before they decided to pick up the phone. We can certainly help to strengthen attachments between these moms and their babies and support the relationships that have been troubled by the months before their desperate calls, but we can't take away the lost moments. And this can be heartbreaking.

So, this goes out to all of you who may be, right at this moment, in that middle zone. To those of you who are reading this book in secret when the lights are out because you don't want anyone else to know that you might not be feeling so well. To those of you who have worked so hard over the last number of months to will this depression or anxiety away only to find it still cuddling up with you at night. To those of you who are so ashamed by how you feel that you would sacrifice your own well-being for secrecy. To those of you who are fantasizing of running away, who are having scary thoughts, or who have thought quietly about how much easier it would be if you simply weren't here but who have not told a soul about any of this.

If this is you, *please reach out to a trained mental health professional!* For you, for your babies, for your partners, for your family and friends, and for those of us on the receiving end of the phone line who are here to help you to feel better. You matter.

Off the Hook

It's about time to take yourself off the hook.

This seems to be the theme of my work with moms so often. Each and every woman who walks into my office in sunny Boulder is challenged at some point with the all-too-common tendency to put limitless amounts of pressure on herself to be a certain way, usually around an idyllic (and very unrealistic) expectation of what it means to be a "perfect mother." You know all about this, I am sure: the pressure to keep the house clean, laundry done, children happy (always), healthy (and homemade) food on the table...the pressure to look good, to be back on the treadmill or in the yoga class and to gain pre-pregnancy fitness now. The pressure to return to work with the same interest and vengeance as before you were pregnant. The pressure to want to stay home with your baby at all times. The pressure to be selfless at all costs. The pressure to have "all your ducks in a row" at each moment, which, quite frankly, is pretty much impossible with one or more little ones around. The pressure to be happy since you have wanted to be a mother for so long.

So, why do we all do this? Why is it so hard to cut ourselves some slack and to realize that we are being "perfect" in all of our "imperfection"? I think it is fair to say that almost every mom looks around her and wonders how "everyone else" is managing so well, when she feels that she is not. Yet, the very moms who are being envied for their "perfection" and "grace" are often those who are next in line for their appointment at my office. They, too, feel as though they are falling apart at the seams.

At some point, giving ourselves a little slack is imperative. The pressure to be a "perfect mother" can drown out the realization that you doing a wonderful job as it is. I would argue that a perfect mother is not she who has a clean house, folded laundry, play dates arranged for a month, and children who never cry. Decades of studies have shown that what matters most in the parent-child relationship is emotional presence, empathy, and attunement, and not logistical beauty. The greatest gift that we can all give to our children is our own happiness and fulfillment, and so I invite you to focus on what really matters to you the most in achieving this. I invite you to let yourself off the hook for the rest.

What it Feels Like to Be a Mack Truck...

...and suddenly come to a full stop after speeding down the highway at about 80 miles an hour.

I can think of no better title for this chapter.

I wonder how many of you can empathize with this particular Mack truck. You have been cruising about in your life. You are an adult and have finally found a way to feel in control of your identity, and you are feeling pretty darn good about yourself. Perhaps you are a professional in one field or another. You have joined many other women in this generation who are making things happen in the world. You are accomplishing. And doing. And moving. And shaking. You are being noticed and validated for your accomplishments. You have expectations of yourself (that come from both within and also from society) to achieve. And you are!

Then you have a baby, and guess what? Suddenly the world seems to stop around you. But this "stopping" is complicated. Some people expect you to simply "slow down" and "be happy at home with your baby." People say you must rest. Stay off your feet. Heal. People encourage you to "just be" for a while. People say "you are so lucky that all you need to do is to be home and stare at your sweet babe!"

Others (perhaps the biggest other in this is yourself) expect you to continue to move. And shake. And do.

Along with the collection of very real and often very uncomfortable emotions that accompany having a baby is the very real and often uncomfortable truth that suddenly "doing" involves being at home in your PJ's all day, ruminating about the color and texture of your kiddo's poop, practicing (and struggling) over and over to get breastfeeding right, practicing (and struggling) to forgive yourself when it's not that easy, and trying, often though trial and error, to understand and connect with this new little being who relies on you for his or her well-being.

Oh, and on top of all that, your hormones and brain chemicals are deciding to rebel against you, and so even if you wanted to "just be" with your baby, it is literally impossible to do so.

Ready, set, STOP!

Ugh...Mack truck-like, no?

While we know that the first layer of risk in developing a postpartum mood disorder is the biochemical imbalance that occurs after giving birth due, mainly, to rampant changes in hormone levels, we also know that other psychological and social risks can exacerbate an already challenging situation. Women who feel more grounded when they are in control, women who set high standards for themselves and live by "perfectionist" thinking, and women who are very, very used to knowing what to expect tend to have a harder time once their babies arrive. In addition, lacking social support (and we are in a society that expects women to do it all by themselves gracefully!), family of origin conflict, and traumatic experiences can all contribute to a new mom's vulnerability.

So, all of this is to say that if you feel like you are suddenly asked to slow down after being so used to moving so quickly, or if you feel like you are expected to do it all even though your body and/or baby is telling you not to, you are absolutely not alone. And if you feel overwhelmed or anxious or sad because you can't seem to feel happy slowing down in this very fast-paced world of ours, you aren't alone either. This transition called "new motherhood" is just plain complicated.

The Postpartum Earthquake

Having a new baby is like a little earthquake, is it not? Everything around you shifts and moves with the birth of that little one. Then, wham, just like that you are needing to reestablish your new relationship to the things in your life—to yourself, your body, your partner/spouse, your family of origin, your friends, your work, your energy levels, your thoughts, and on and on. And many of us are not prepared for this sudden loss of grounding. It can feel like we are lost in our own surroundings, especially after we have known ourselves and how we fit into the world around us for so long. This can be extremely overwhelming.

A few things might be helpful along the way toward regaining comfort in your new relationship to things, whether it's your new relationship with yourself, other people in your life, or your environment. This is always a process, of course, because nothing happens overnight. But a new acceptance and understanding can certainly occur with thought and support.

1. What are your wellness priorities *right now?* In other words, what three things do you know you need to feel healthy and well? Not what 10 or 20 things, but what three? I'm asking about *right now*—not a week or a year from now or last week or last year. Is sleep important? Eating well? Time outside? Time with your partner? Time with friends? Simply time away? A hot shower? Exercise? Getting dressed each morning? A hug? Writing these three things down and then putting them somewhere that you can see them regularly can be helpful. When you are drawn to cleaning the house, doing laundry, or returning emails, ask yourself where these things lie on your current priority list. If they aren't there, consider replacing your time at that moment with something that is.
2. Ask yourself what *your* definition of a "good *enough*" or "perfect *enough*" mother is. Not what your own mom, or your friends, or the people who have given you their two cents, or the piles of books on your bedside table might say. What do *you* want to incorporate into your role as mom? Again, consider writing these things down and look at them each night. Ask yourself what you did that day or how you were that day in relation to this list. I would bet that you are doing more and being more from your list than you think you are.
3. What are the "shoulds" that you are holding so tightly onto? We all have them. In other words, what are the expectations—society's or your own—that you are focusing time and energy on? Are these expectations realistic, or are they myths?
4. Do you need to say goodbye to parts of your life? If so, sometimes going

through a real mourning process around this is important and useful. It is completely understandable and valid that you might feel regret at what you are suddenly needing to give up, be it more time to yourself, expectation, control, spontaneity, work, intimacy with your partner, ideas about your body, etc. The truth is that these parts of your life will emerge again if you want them to and when time allows. I had a friend recently ask me how, as women and mothers, we can possibly "do it all"—how can we be good at our work, present with our kids and partners, keep up with the news, read books, keep a clean house, plant a garden, exercise, travel, stay in touch, smell the flowers...? My answer to her is that we can do all of those things if we choose to. Just not all at the same time.

5. Three can feel like a crowd. Especially at first. You and your partner may have planned for this baby and maybe even worked at conceiving for a while. But it can certainly feel like a balanced pair suddenly became unglued when a third party needs love, care, and attention all the time. Even if you feel like you know your partner better than anyone else in the world, you do not necessarily know who he or she is as a parent. You really can't possibly know who you will be as a parent either until you are one. So, taking some time to get to know your partner—and yourself—*again* is important. And remember, of course, that while you are both the same people, you will also learn many, many new things along the way.

The thing about earthquakes is that surroundings can feel, and look, destroyed for a while. It can suddenly seem as though nothing is recognizable. But with time and often effort, things get rebuilt, they grow back, and life returns to a "*new* normal."

Yours will too!

Ever Wonder Where You Went?

It's this crazy thing: You have a baby and suddenly become a mother and then, either immediately or months or years later, you think, "Wait a second, where did I go? Where is that person I know myself to be?" This can, for many women, feel like missing an old friend.

When we become mothers, we change, undoubtedly. We grow. We develop. We learn, albeit not always happily, about the importance of resetting expectations and about the need to be flexible.

But becoming a mother does not mean that you have lost yourself. It is certainly true that for many women, a process of mourning the loss of previous lives is incredibly important and healing. At the same time, I am suggesting that **You** are still **You**—that your truest self still exists but is just buried underneath all of the change.

So, for those of you who are feeling that you aren't entirely sure how to reconnect with your core, I suggest you find a pen, make yourself comfortable with a cup of tea and a quiet house (yes, you might need to wait until the time is right for this), and tap back into your "Moments of Grace." This exercise will take about 15 minutes.

> STEP 1: On a blank piece of paper, list all of the moments or times in your life when you felt like your "best self." These can be as large and encompassing as a stage in life such as high school, senior year in college, or during your pregnancy and as small and specific as the feeling in a hot shower after being out in the cold. And anywhere in between. There is no "right" or "wrong" here, and the idea is to tap into those times in your life when you felt *present* and *alive.*
>
> STEP 2: For each of the items in your list above, write down words that describe each experience. These words will most likely be adjectives, but they don't need to be. In other words, what are the *qualities* of these moments that made them so special. Most likely, you will find some repetition.
>
> STEP 3: If you have more than five or six words in your list from above, circle about five or six that resonate most with you. Write these in a separate list.

These words, Dear Readers, represent your *core values*—the pieces of yourself that make you who you are. They are still here.

The trick now is to find ways in your current life to access these qualities. If you really think about it, are you doing some things now that encompass these values? If not, what is getting in your way: unrealistic expectations, fear, self-doubt, or guilt? Can you "think outside of the box" and reset expectations so you are able to make choices that will involve some of these values?

This is not easy stuff, I know. Many of you might be thinking, "*Yeah, but I am a mom now, so I can't go traveling and explore the world so as to tap into my values of adventure and exploration*!"

My suggestion, if this is you, is to think about whether or not your thinking is focused on what you *aren't* doing, rather than what you *are*.

When you have tapped back into yourself, take a moment to recognize this and silently tell yourself "Welcome Home."

And This Is What I Know

1. Every mom who walks into my office is there because she is a great mom... even if she can't see it yet.
2. Motherhood is hard for 99.9999 percent of women (and I'd really be interested to meet that special 0.0001 percent who finds it easy). Those moms you see who you think are "perfect" are no more perfect than you are.
3. Everyone who seeks help for a postpartum mood disorder by a trained and appropriate provider, and who follows through with treatment recommendations, does get well.
4. Suffering from postpartum depression/postpartum anxiety is devastating and feels like it will never end.
5. With help, it does.
6. Your baby needs you.
7. You deserve to take breaks, even if you think that you do not.
8. This motherhood thing is, most likely, not what you expected.
9. You feel like you have lost yourself, but you have not. You are still you.
10. If you are suffering from a postpartum mood disorder like PPD, you are scared.
11. A time is coming when you will no longer be as scared as you are now.
12. You are not alone, even if you feel that you are. Millions of women are suffering just like you are. You are part of an army.
13. Your sadness, anxiety, uncertainty, apathy, hopelessness, irritability, regret, immobility, difficulty concentrating, overwhelm, and despair are not character flaws. These things do not define you. They are just symptoms of your postpartum mood disorder, and as you heal, these symptoms will go away.
14. Your partner wants desperately to see you well, and their withdrawal, frustration, impatience, or inability to empathize is most likely due to their uncertainty about what you need from them to feel better.
15. Underneath all of the advice, opinion, and judgment that exists, you absolutely know what is best for you. You are your own expert.
16. No one parenting philosophy is better than the next. What matters most is what works for each individual family.
17. Your little one will be happy if you are happy. Take care of you.

18. We are coming together—all of us—in one great, huge effort to spread awareness about PPD and other postpartum mood disorders. You are a part of this effort, and we need you.
19. You are human. You are allowed to make mistakes.
20. The more you try to control the things in your life that you cannot, the more anxious you will become. This is simply the way it goes.
21. Letting go of the above is much easier said than done. But it is possible.
22. Your baby is not fussy because he/she doesn't like you or thinks that you are a bad mom. Your baby is fussy because he/she is a baby. That little one doesn't know any more than you do what he/she needs most of the time.
23. You are doing the best you can.
24. You love your baby even if you do not love much about being a mom right now. Those two things can absolutely come hand in hand.
25. You are a teacher. Along this journey, you will teach your family, your friends, your children, and your community what it means to be human. People will grow through knowing you.
26. Everything that I say is easier said from my chair than from yours.

What I See That You May Not

Most days in my psychotherapy office are marked by many, many tears. I see so much shame. So much disappointment. So much guilt. So much embarrassment. The moms in my office have felt let down by themselves. They have felt lost. They are afraid of failing. They are unsure about almost everything. The moms in my office have (understandably) wondered *"Why me?"* and *"What am I doing wrong?"* and "*Why can't I do this when everyone else can?"* The last place these moms ever expected to be during their first year with a new baby is in my office. With a box of tissues in their laps.

While these women will remain anonymous, this note goes out to them. And to others who may feel similar to the mamas above. This note goes out to you because, although I know that each one of you feels insignificant and lost and incompetent, I see a much different picture.

So, moms, listen loud and clear:

You are beautiful. You are wise. You are significant and needed and valuable. You are fabulous mothers simply for taking the initiative to be in my office or someone else's. You are competent and strong and skilled and conscientious even if you do not feel that way. You are deserving. You are "perfect enough!" You are human. You are absolutely allowed to struggle and waver and be unsure and not know. In fact, you are all the more real for feeling all of the things that you are brave enough to acknowledge.

Your children are lucky to have you.

A day will come when you recognize all of this. Even if you aren't there yet.

You Can't Stop the Waves, But You Can Learn How to Surf

The title of this chapter comes from Jon Kabat-Zinn, who is the founder of mindfulness-based stress reduction (MBSR). He teaches the use of mindfulness meditation as a technique to help people cope with stress, anxiety, and pain. "You can't stop the waves, but you can learn how to surf." I find these words to be hugely fitting when thinking about the wonderful yet often chaotic journey of motherhood. This is why they are found on the very first page of my website. If you are a surfer, you will know exactly what this phrase means, and if you are not, let me explain.

Picture this: It's a beautiful day at the beach (maybe you are in San Francisco, or Mexico, or Bali, or some other wonderful location), and the ocean is vibrant and blue. You decide to take out a surfboard and paddle around for a while. You have always wanted to surf. From the shore, the waves look beautiful. Yet when you are out past your comfort zone, they begin to feel a little less tame. One after another, the waves come toward you. You get tossed and turned in the white water, your board bobbing alongside, behind, or in front of you—or on top of you if you aren't careful. Your heart begins to race. You swallow water as each new wave breaks. It is calm for a few moments, and you scramble on top of your surfboard again, this time holding on for dear life as you see another set of waves coming your way. You close your eyes, or pray, or imagine yourself somewhere else. Whatever it takes to get through this next series of waves. It goes on and on as you become more exhausted, depleted, and scared. You feel as though you can't catch your breath. Because those waves just keep coming.

Or, you can learn how to surf.

Once you do, what felt scary is now glorious. Yeah, you have those moments when a big wave comes through and catches you off guard, but for the most part you take it in stride. You understand the rhythms of the ocean, and so you are more able to predict what is coming. You have your timing down, so you welcome each wave with a grace that comes from within. It comes from your core. It comes from your balance. You move with the wave instead of fighting it. You paddle along with it until you catch its momentum, and you stand. Tall. You feel exhilarated and brave and proud. The wave carries you along until it dumps you safely on the beach. And then you turn around and go out for more...you battle the breaking waves until you are past that initial fear, and you are ready to catch the next ride. Perhaps bigger and more challenging than the last.

In motherhood, you must learn how to surf. Those waves just keep on coming, anyway.

Once you do that, you can begin to move forward with an authenticity and a pace that will lead you in the direction you desire.

What If Supermom Was You?

Work with me for a moment here.

If you believed that you had the capacity to keep going even when you were scared, to love yourself even when you were messy and unorganized, to heal little hearts simply by being you, exactly as you are, and to be a role model to the world by trusting yourself and your deepest wisdom, what would you do differently?

Really. Right now. What would you do differently?

Would you take a deep breath? Call for support? Look at yourself tenderly in the mirror? Drink some water or go for a walk or gaze at the blue of the sky? Would you lean toward health? Would you, even if briefly, feel powerful?

You see, therein lies the soul of a Supermom: She believes in herself.

Yeah, I know, she dons that badass outfit, but it's not the outfit that makes her, *her*! It's what is inside of it, under the skin, close to her heart.

We make up these stories about ourselves all the time: *I'm not good enough. I'm too weak. I don't know how. I'm not worthy. I'm a bad mother.*

Stories. That's all they are. Those stories are the bad guys. Between you and me? They actually aren't that smart. They just aren't real.

But a Supermom is *definitely* real. And she is *you*.

Because you are doing it. Right now. You are reading this book and taking a breath and getting up in the morning. You might be struggling and exhausted and scared and lonely, but you are doing it. Still.

Hi there Supermom.

It's your bravery to keep going. Your tender heart that has its moment every once in a while, even though it is protective and sharp a lot of the time. Your quiet knowing deep underneath all the uncertainty is Wonder Woman telling you what she knows. From deep inside of *you*.

That is where a Supermom lives.

She is you.

You are her.

Just start paying attention. You will see.

BOOK RESOURCES

General Postpartum Support

POSTPARTUM SUPPORT INTERNATIONAL (PSI)
www.postpartum.net

PSI Helpline

1-800-944-4773

Text "Help" to 800-944-4773 (EN)

Text en Español: 971-203-7773

MGH CENTER FOR WOMEN'S MENTAL HEALTH: REPRODUCTIVE PSYCHIATRY RESOURCES & INFORMATION CENTER
https://womensmentalhealth.org

SELENI INSTITUTE
https://www.seleni.org

POSTPARTUM STRESS CENTER
https://postpartumstress.com/

POSTPARTUM SUPPORT CENTER
https://www.postpartumsc.org

HRSA: MATERNAL & CHILD HEALTH
https://mchb.hrsa.gov

NATIONAL MATERNAL MENTAL HEALTH HOTLINE
1-833-9-HELP4MOMS (1-833-943-5746)

General Support Groups and Therapists

PSI DIRECTORY
https://www.psidirectory.com

PSI - ONLINE SUPPORT GROUPS - includes support groups for PMADs, BIPOC and LGBTQ+ individuals, dads, parents of children with disabilities, grief and loss, military moms, and more
https://www.postpartum.net/get-help/psi-online-support-meetings/

PSI - FIND LOCAL SUPPORT
https://www.postpartum.net/get-help/locations/

POSTPARTUM DEPRESSION SUPPORT GROUPS IN THE U.S. & CANADA:
https://postpartumprogress.com/ppd-support-groups-in-the-u-s-canada

POSTPARTUM DEPRESSION TREATMENT PROGRAMS AND SPECIALISTS:
https://postpartumprogress.com/
womens-mental-health-treatment-programs-specialists-us-canada-australia

Postpartum Mood & Anxiety Disorders (PMADs)

BOOKS:
Dropping the Baby and Other Scary Thoughts, by Karen Kleiman, Amy Wenzel, Hilary Waller, and Abby Adler Mandel, (Routledge, 2020).

The Pregnancy and Postpartum Anxiety Workbook: Practical Skills to Help You Overcome Anxiety, Worry, Panic Attacks, Obsessions, and Compulsions, by Pamela S. Wiegartz and Kevin L. Gyoerkoe (New Harbinger Publications, 2009).

The Postpartum Depression Workbook: Strategies to Overcome Negative Thoughts, Calm Stress, and Improve Your Mood, by Abigail Burd (Rockridge Press; 2020)

Trauma

BIRTH TRAUMA ASSOCIATION (BTA)
https://www.birthtraumaassociation.org.uk

LOVE FOR LILLY – NICU SUPPORT
https://www.loveforlily.org

PREGNANT SURVIVORS
https://pregnantsurvivors.org

PREVENTION & TREATMENT OF TRAUMATIC CHILDBIRTH (PATTCH)
https://pattch.org

[Book] *When Survivors Give Birth* by Penny Simkin & Phyllis Klaus

Grief & Infant/Child/Neonatal Loss

GLOW IN THE WOODS
www.glowinthewoods.com

COMPASSIONATE FRIENDS
https://www.compassionatefriends.org

MARCH OF DIMES
https://www.marchofdimes.org/complications/dealing-with-grief-after-the-death-of-your-baby.aspx

MISCARRIAGE MATTERS
https://www.mymiscarriagematters.org

RETURN TO ZERO
https://rtzhope.org

SHARE
https://nationalshare.org

STAR LEGACY FOUNDATION
https://starlegacyfoundation.org

SUPPORT FOR LOSS AND GRIEF IN PREGNANCY AND POSTPARTUM
https://www.postpartum.net/get-help/loss-grief-in-pregnancy-postpartum/

Abortion Support

EXHALE - SUPPORT FOLLOWING AN ABORTION
https://exhaleprovoice.org

AFTER ABORTION HOTLINE
Call 617-749-2948 Or Text "Exhale Pro-Voice"

Dads

POSTPARTUM SUPPORT FOR DADS
https://www.postpartum.net/get-help/help-for-dads/

CENTER FOR MEN'S EXCELLENCE
https://www.menexcel.com

DADDIT (REDDIT GROUP)
https://www.reddit.com/r/daddit/

MISCARRIAGE FOR MEN
https://www.miscarriageformen.com

HOW DAD'S CAN BUILD A NETWORK OF PARENTING ALLIES AT WORK
https://hbr.org/2021/08/how-dads-can-build-a-network-of-parenting-allies-at-work

Adoption

ADOPTING.ORG

WHO TO TALK TO ABOUT ADOPTION DEPRESSION?
https://adopting.org/talk-about-adoption-depression/

NATIONAL COUNCIL FOR ADOPTION (NCFA)

UNDERSTANDING PARENTAL POSTADOPTION DEPRESSION (PPD)
https://adoptioncouncil.org/publications/understanding-parental-postadoption-depression/

SUPPORT FOR ADOPTIVE AND SUPPORT MOMS
https://www.postpartum.net/get-help/adoptive-and-birth-mothers/

Infertility & Reproductive Medicine

AMERICAN SOCIETY FOR REPRODUCTIVE MEDICINE (ASRM):
www.asrm.org

RESOLVE: THE NATIONAL INFERTILITY ASSOCIATION
https://resolve.org

COPING WITH SECONDARY INFERTILITY
https://www.seleni.org/advice-support/2018/2/28/coping-with-secondary-infertility

MINDFULNESS DURING IVF
https://www.seleni.org/advice-support/2018/2/28/mindfulness-during-ivf

Working Mothers

CHAMBER OF MOTHERS
https://www.chamberofmothers.com

MAMATTORNEY - LEGAL SUPPORT FOR WORKING MOTHERS
https://www.themamattorney.com

WORKING MOMS AGAINST GUILT
www.workingmomsagainstguilt.com

LGBTQ+ Families

SUPPORT FOR QUEER AND TRANS FAMILIES
https://www.postpartum.net/get-help/queer-parents/

RETURN TO ZERO: LGBTQIA+
https://rtzhope.org/lgbtq

LGBT PREGNANCY LOSS INFORMATION SHEET (AUSTRALIAN PHYCOLOGICAL SOCIETY)
https://psychology.org.au/getmedia/9ea8dd55-7c2b-4653-8371-b1f732b70b58/lgbt_pregnancy_loss.pdf

[BOOK] *Reproductive Losses: Challenges to LGBTQ Family-Making,* by Christa Craven (Routledge, Taylor & Francis Group, 2019).

BIPOC Mothers/Parents

BLACK MAMAS MATTER ALLIANCE
https://blackmamasmatter.org

SHADES OF BLUE PROJECT
https://www.shadesofblueproject.org

MATER MEA BLOG
https://www.matermea.com

MELINATED MOMS COMMUNITY
https://melinatedmoms.com

LOVELAND FOUNDATION & FUND
https://thelovelandfoundation.org

BLACK EMOTIONAL AND MENTAL HEALTH COLLECTIVE (BEAM)
https://beam.community

Military Families

SUPPORT FOR MILITARY FAMILIES
https://www.postpartum.net/get-help/military-families/

UNITED STATES MARINE CORPS

https://www.usmc-mccs.org/services/family/new-parent-support-program/

U.S. ARMY'S PARENTHOOD, PREGNANCY AND POSTPARTUM DIRECTIVE
https://www.army.mil/article/255884/soldiers_inspire_new_army_directive_on_parenthood_pregnancy_and_postpartum_policies

Medication & Alternative Treatments

MASSACHUSETTS GENERAL HOSPITAL'S CENTER FOR WOMEN'S HEALTH:
https://womensmentalhealth.org/specialty-clinics/breastfeeding-and-psychiatric-medication/

PRESCRIPTION MEDICATION USE WHILE BREASTFEEDING
https://www.cdc.gov/breastfeeding/breastfeeding-special-circumstances/vaccinations-medications-drugs/prescription-medication-use.html

BREASTFEEDING AND MEDICATIONS: WHAT'S SAFE?
https://www.mayoclinic.org/healthy-lifestyle/infant-and-toddler-health/in-depth/breastfeeding-and-medications/art-20043975

Meditation & Mindfulness

APPS:
Calm: www.calm.com

Insight Timer: https://insighttimer.com

Mindful Mamas: https://app.mindfulmamasclub.com/

Expectant: https://expectful.com

JKZ Meditations (Guided Mindfulness Meditation Practices with Jon Kabat-Zinn):

www.mindfulnesscds.com

[BOOK] *Expecting Mindfully: Nourish Your Emotional Well-Being and Prevent Depression During Pregnancy and Postpartum* by Sona Dimidjian, PhD, and Sherryl H Goodman, PhD

ACKNOWLEDGMENTS

When things are done well, they are done within the context of community. When I sit down to write, I often wonder where all of my creative thinking comes from. I am amazed when it flows from someplace outside of me. It certainly is not all mine. For years, I have been a sponge as a learner; there are never enough podcasts, inspirational books, or important courses in which I can participate. I often feel like I just can't get enough. So, this book is a creation that requires a tribute to many of my mentors, big and small, near and far, aware and unaware of my total appreciation of them. They include: Pema Chodron, Sarah Blondin, Elizabeth Gilbert, Jonathan Fields, Thich Nhat Hahn, Deepak Chopra, Byron Katie, Diana Chapman, Kelly Wendorf, Eckhart Tolle, Bronnie Ware, Oprah Winfrey, Diego Perez, Kristin Neff, Glennon Doyle, and the many unnamed mentors whose podcasts and books I devour.

In addition, my closer network of colleagues, partners, and mentors has undoubtedly helped me to pull all of this together with grace and enthusiasm. Thank you to Karen Kleiman, Wendy Davis, Emily Horowitz, Amy Slaymaker, Jennifer Cunningham, Marie Galastro, Julie Solomon, and Cathy Heller. You all play a significant role in my professional journey.

To the community of women in my life who are excited by my excitement. There is no bigger gift in a friendship. You know who you are.

To the village of mothers who are always there to help support my role as a working mom with carpools, parenting support, last-minute sleepovers for my girls, humor, and encouragement. Motherhood is not meant to be done alone, and you all make it possible for me to mother both my children and myself well.

To my husband, Jamie. There is nobody else I would rather parent with. Thank you for your part in making me a mother.

Finally, there is no birth of a mother without important people in both directions. I happen to have the incredible honor of sitting in between women of whom I am in awe. To my late mom, Margaret Lawson Shaw, who gave me infinite love and taught me to trust myself always. I think of her every second that I mother my own daughters. This book, and the direct work I do with mothers, is in honor of her. And to my two biggest teachers—my daughters, Kinley and Bridger. You force me to be a better me. Thank you for being you, just as you are. I love watching you become.

And in between those women is me. I want to share gratitude for the parts of me that have learned and committed to mothering myself well. That has been the biggest lesson of all.

My heart is full.

ABOUT THE AUTHOR

Kate Kripke, LCSW, PMH-C is an author, thought leader, psychotherapist, consultant, and coach with a specialty in maternal mental health. She is the Founding Director of The Postpartum Wellness Center in Boulder, Colorado, where she provides direct clinical support to mothers. Outside of her clinical practice, Kate actively engages with the larger community of mothers through her virtual coaching and consulting support.

Kate lives in Boulder, Colorado, with her husband, two amazing daughters, and dog Darwin. She can be found taking care of herself while hiking at Sanitas, spending time with her girlfriends, absorbing herself in a podcast or book, sitting quietly in nature, and having dance parties in the kitchen (sometimes completely by herself).

Learn more at www.katekripke.com and www.pwcboulder.com.